grit AND GRACE

FIGHTING BREAST CANCER
ONE STEP AT A TIME

Carrie S. Bell

CARRIE S. BELL

Grit and Grace: Fighting Breast Cancer One Step at a Time
Copyright © 2014 by Carrie S. Bell

For information about this title or to order other books and/or electronic media, contact the publisher:
Better Health Books
Scottsdale, AZ
www.carriesbell.com
betterhealthbooks@gmail.com

Library of Congress Control Number: 2014936531
ISBN:
978-0-9960476-0-9 (print)
978-0-9960476-1-6 (e-book)
Printed in the United States of America
Cover and Interior design by: 1106 Design

Publisher's Cataloging-In-Publication Data
Bell, Carrie S.
    Grit and grace: fighting breast cancer one step at a time / Carrie S. Bell. — 1st ed.
    1. Memoir 2. Breast cancer 3. Health 4. Inspiration.

For my husband Moe Bell, with love and gratitude

CONTENTS

PREFACE

I'm the neighbor woman you see passing on the sidewalk, coaching kids in the park, or pushing a cart down the aisles of the supermarket. I'm the mom who volunteers at your children's school, the lady in your office, or a member of your book club. I'm a wife, mother, daughter, sister, and friend. I don't have a famous name or face, but you know me. Chances are I'm a lot like you or someone you love.

A few years ago I got breast cancer. Like so many women diagnosed with the disease, I had no known risk factors. I'd been healthy all my life and had lived an intentionally healthy lifestyle. I could not have been more surprised to learn that I had cancer. At first my tumor seemed small and localized, but further investigation revealed more extensive disease that would require the full arsenal of cancer treatments. To help me process what was happening and stay in touch with loved ones, I created a blog about my treatment experience. At the urging of friends and family, I'm sharing what I wrote during that time, plus some postscripts penned more recently. My goal is to provide insight and inspiration for other breast cancer patients. Life goes on during treatment, and it's not all bad.

To each person fighting this disease, I wish the best possible medical care, a tidal wave of love and support from your "village," a wealth of wisdom that can only be gained through adversity, and that you will find specks of joy to keep you going when you feel hopeless and sad.

"You're doing this with grit and grace, Carrie," a friend said during my cancer treatment. Thank you, Eilene, for one of the nicest compliments I've ever received—and for the perfect title for this book.

ACKNOWLEDGMENTS

Gratitude is the foundation of a good life. I am grateful to everyone who helped me survive breast cancer and also to those who encouraged me to produce *Grit and Grace*.

Without the persistent urging of my husband, Moe Bell, this book never would have become a reality. Sometimes he knows what is best for me before I do. Thanks, Moe, for pushing me just enough, but not too much.

I'm also indebted to three friends who gave of their time to read my manuscript in its entirety. Without doubt, their feedback made the book better:

I barely knew Roy Skogstrom before sending him my book, but now I consider him a friend for life. Thanks, Roy, for the comments, questions, unwavering support, sick jokes, and of course, the commas. You are the Comma King!

Gayle Nobel has long inspired me with her example as an author and as someone who faces life's challenges with courage and optimism. Thanks, Gayle, for being in my corner as I assembled the manuscript. Your positive response helped me to overcome my doubts and move forward.

Barclay Schraff listened to my concerns about this book during weekly hikes for over a year. Always, she knew the right questions to ask. Thanks, Barclay, for your patience, encouragement, and helpful insights on the trail and as a "reader."

I am also grateful to others who provided a sounding board for me during the creation of *Grit and Grace*. Special thanks to Pam Tomlinson, Melissa Abraham, Angie Stenberg, Emily Bell, Brian Bell, Mary Ann Rowland, and the Scottsdale Writers' Critique Group.

Finally, I'd like to thank Michele DeFilippo, Ronda Rawlins, and the team at 1106 Design for their good cheer and high standards in the design and production of this book.

DIAGNOSIS

"Believe in yourself and all that you are. Know that there is something inside you that is greater than any obstacle."

—Christian D. Larson

Introduction

August 2011

I am a fifty-two-year-old woman whose life was changed forever on August 15, 2011, when I was diagnosed with breast cancer. Only a month ago I had hopes that my healthy lifestyle would help me live to be 100. Now I'm a cancer patient facing months of chemotherapy to be followed by surgery and radiation. All of this will be necessary to defeat my aggressive disease. I still want to live to a ripe old age—to see my children mature, to know their kids, and to find out what life will teach me as I grow old. Though I'll fight with every bit of my strength to remain among the living, I understand now that there are no guarantees for anyone. Life is a precious gift and I'm appreciating each day like never before.

How I Found My Cancer

Everyone has been asking how my cancer was discovered. It all started last February. I was soaping my left armpit in the shower and felt a tiny lump. My physician husband, Moe, thought it was probably a reactive lymph node. "Let's watch it for a month and see if it goes away," he said.

When it didn't disappear, I made an appointment with the nurse practitioner at my OBGYN's office. I saw her in March, and she too believed the lump to be a lymph node. To cover all bases, she wrote me a prescription for a mammogram and an ultrasound of the lump.

On April 6, I had the tests. The mammogram showed nothing. The ultrasound technician called in the radiologist on duty to look at images of the lump on an electronic monitor. The doctor rolled the ultrasound device back and forth over the tiny mass and finally decided he could see a thread connecting it to a larger lymph node. "If I couldn't see that thread, I would stick a needle in it," he said. His report recommended another ultrasound in six months.

I breathed a sigh of relief and continued preparations for a once-in-a-lifetime family trip coming up in July. Over the next few months, I continued to feel the lump. Though it didn't seem any bigger, its presence nagged at the back of my mind. When we returned from vacation, Moe and I agreed I should have another ultrasound to make sure the lump was nothing.

We went for the test on August 12. This time a different radiologist entered the room and had a different conclusion. "This is breast tissue and not a lymph node," she said. "I think we should do a needle biopsy." She did the biopsy right then. Afterward she told me the lump was very tiny. "I do a lot of these biopsies and I rate them 'mildly concerning,' 'moderately concerning,' and 'suspicious.' I would call this one mildly concerning."

Despite her reassuring words and Moe's certainty the lump would be benign, I felt anxious all weekend. When the radiologist called on Monday morning August 15, I hoped it was to tell me I had nothing to worry about. Instead, she informed me I had a 6mm cancerous tumor. Though the cancer was Grade 3, the most aggressive type, the tumor was as tiny as they come. "You have caught this early and have every reason to expect the best outcome," she said.

I was so stunned it was hard to concentrate on the rest of her words.

How I Told My Friends

This is the message I sent to family and friends shortly after my diagnosis, and it's a true story:

August 16, 2011

A nicely dressed young woman rang our doorbell a few minutes ago. She was going door to door to raise $2,300 to participate in the Susan G. Komen 3-Day Walk for the Cure. What timing. She had no way of knowing that I was diagnosed with breast cancer just yesterday. I didn't tell her, but listened as she explained that her grandmother and two aunts had battled the disease.

At a time when the reality of my situation is sinking in, it felt as though the young woman was delivering a message. I am not alone. One in eight women gets diagnosed with breast cancer, and they (or I guess I should say "we") have legions of family members, friends and health care professionals supporting them (us). Moe stood at the door with me as the young lady made her pitch. We exchanged a look and he ran to get his wallet. How strange life is sometimes. I'm pretty sure there will be a 3-Day Walk in my future.

This is my way of telling you about my diagnosis. The tumor is very small and we hope to banish it for good on the first try. I am trying to stay calm and upbeat, though this is all pretty new and scary.

Sometimes Things Get Worse Before They Get Better

Another message to loved ones, explaining things were more complicated than we thought:

August 26, 2011

Hi Everyone,

It has been a mind-bending two weeks. Needle biopsy on August 12, breast cancer diagnosis on August 15, MRI on August 19, call from my surgeon on August 23 to share MRI results suggesting my cancer was far more serious than we first thought. Finding out I had cancer was like a kick in the stomach. Learning it was worse than expected was akin to a body slam from a sumo wrestler. How could this be?

The past several days have involved consultations with various doctors and MRI experts. The problem and blessing of an MRI is that it's so sensitive it picks up everything. What looks like "something" may be real or could be "nothing." Moe tracked down the top MRI guru at Scottsdale Healthcare to help us figure out what was real and what was exaggerated on my MRI. His reading of my situation was less alarming than the original report.

The consensus among my doctors is that I have Stage II or Stage III cancer in the breast and a few lymph nodes. It is invasive ductal cell carcinoma Grade 3, a very aggressive type of cancer, but also one that responds best to chemotherapy. Traditionally, breast cancer is treated with surgery first, followed by chemo, but in my case the doctors feel it is best to reverse the order. The most important thing now is to prevent the cancer from spreading elsewhere, and chemo is the best tool for that job. So, I start treatment next Wednesday. Surgery will follow in about six months, then radiation. It'll be a long journey, but I plan to cross the finish line cancer-free.

Back to the question, "How could this be?" As far as I knew, I had very few risk factors for this disease. No family history of breast cancer, healthy lifestyle, healthy weight, nonsmoker, exercise nut. My only risk factors were having my first child after age thirty, dense breasts, and drinking one glass of wine in the evening.

The diagnosis seemed random until I spoke with the oncologist. His eyebrows rose when I told him about a strong family history of prostate cancer (my father, his two brothers and my paternal grandfather). Apparently, there's a genetic link in some families between prostate cancer in males, and breast and ovarian cancers in females. My blood is being tested to see whether I have the BRCA1 or BRCA2 gene. If your parent has one of the genes, you have a one in two chance of getting one of these cancers. I hope I don't have either gene, but it would answer the question, "Why me?"

As you might imagine, this has been a trying time for our family. I don't know which was worse, waiting for test results or getting the news. At times Moe and I have been overwhelmed by fear and sadness, feelings we have tried to hide from our children, twenty-year-old Brian and Emily, seventeen. So far they seem appropriately concerned but not freaked out. The love and support of family and friends have really helped to lift us up. Thank you so much for your phone calls, e-mails, texts, and prayers. Please keep them coming. It feels good to have a treatment plan, but there will be challenging times ahead. I'd be a liar if I didn't admit to being scared.

Postscript: The day we received that MRI report was one of the worst of my life. I had been out shopping that afternoon trying to cheer myself up, but compulsively wondering how shirts I was trying on would fit after surgery, and whether I would be able to wear anything sleeveless once lymph nodes had been carved out of my armpit. With my future so uncertain, why was I even buying new clothes? I forced myself to stuff those negative thoughts and shop on.

When I came in the door just after 5 p.m., my husband was waiting for me with a drawn face and bloodshot eyes. The elevator in my gut plunged to the bottom floor. "What's wrong?" I said.

Moe hugged me tightly before delivering the bad news. That afternoon he had read my MRI report on the hospital website (I had given my permission beforehand.) It suggested a 5 cm tumor in my left breast and involvement of at least two lymph nodes. As we went over the findings, I realized I could well die from this cancer. That awareness has been with me every day since, though I try not to dwell on it. Staying "in the moment," fully occupied with whatever I'm doing, seems to help.

CHEMOTHERAPY

2

"It's not the load that breaks you down, it's the way you carry it."

—Lou Holtz

First Chemo

Tuesday, September 13, 2011

I had my first chemotherapy infusion on Friday, September 2. It was supposed to have happened two days earlier but had to be postponed for insurance reasons. On Friday morning, I went to the hospital five minutes from my home to have a "Power Port" catheter installed in my chest. The port is a little chunk of plastic and metal that sits just under the skin on the right side of my chest. There is a black Frankenstein scar running beneath it, where an incision has been glued together, in case I need reminding that the port is there. A little tube connected to the port snakes over my clavicle and down into a vein next to my heart. All of my chemo infusions will go through the Power Port, which leaves my much-poked arm veins breathing sighs of relief.

The Power Port worked beautifully on Friday afternoon, when a nurse in my oncologist's chemo suite hooked up an IV bag to it and let the cancer-killing fluids flow in. My first four infusions will be a combination of Adriamycin and Cytoxan. The last four infusions will contain a different drug, Taxol. If all goes well (i.e., my white blood cell count stays high enough and I'm not too sick), I will get chemo every two weeks for four months. The oncologist has already said okay to a week off in October to allow us to take a family trip to San Diego, so the whole process could take a little longer.

Chemo isn't painful, though I could feel the liquid flowing into my chest. Mostly, I felt like a science experiment. It was strange to sit there for two hours while toxins that could save my life entered my body. I went from someone on no medications to major junkie. I took an anti-nausea medication called Emend right before the infusion and two other anti-nausea pills (Ondansetron and Dexamethasone) with dinner afterward. I was told to keep taking these pills for two days after chemo.

Despite the meds, I was nauseated within two hours of finishing chemo and dry heaving off and on all evening. One of the meds knocked me out enough to let me sleep most of Friday night. On Saturday morning, I tried to eat and drink and take my pills, but nothing stayed down. This went on until about 2 p.m., when I started to feel a bit better. I was recovered enough by 3 to go to the hospital for a shot (Neulasta) to boost my white blood cell count, standard procedure the day after chemo.

Though my head felt a bit foggy and I couldn't eat normally for a few more days, I saw improvement every day. I was walking in the park by Monday and hiking up a mountain by Thursday (this worried my husband, but was great for my spirits). I have been more tired than usual and had a low white blood cell count the Friday after chemo, but have been otherwise very encouraged by how my body has responded.

So far, this is nothing I can't handle. Another shot in the arm on Friday boosted my white count to superhuman levels by Monday afternoon, which means I will be able to have my next infusion this

Friday morning. I know it sounds twisted, but this makes me very happy. Bring on the cancer killers!

Postscript: In the first weeks after diagnosis, focusing on facts and descriptions was my default. Somewhere in my subconscious, I probably thought that if I could understand what was happening to me physically, I'd be able to deal with it emotionally.

Though I couldn't yet put words to my inner turmoil, there were times when it threatened to overwhelm me. At my first doctor's appointment after the MRI, I paced the waiting room, unable to sit still, read a magazine, or concentrate on anything. My mouth was dry, my pulse raced, and I felt every heartbeat pounding inside my head. I remember thinking: *This is what it feels like to be jumping out of your skin.*

I tried to calm myself by taking deep breaths, but when the nurse took my blood pressure it was the highest it's ever been. I was a fit hiker, but felt like I might have a stroke at any minute. Only the warm, matter-of-fact words of my breast surgeon managed to ease my distress. She'd seen cases like mine before, and thought we had a good chance of stopping the spread of my cancer with chemo. As she presented my options, I hung on her every word and absorbed her positive energy.

"Everybody says chemo is the worst part, and you'll get that out of the way first," the surgeon said, smiling. "The rest will seem easy after that."

When Moe and I left her building, my head no longer throbbed and I breathed a little easier. *Just maybe, I'll get through this,* I thought.

Hair, or the Lack Thereof

Wednesday, September 14, 2011

Before starting chemotherapy, I learned that most patients lose their hair three to four weeks after the first treatment. Along with prescriptions for multiple pills, my oncologist gave me one on which he had written "cranial prosthesis." That's the fancy term for "wig." Those of you who know me well can imagine my reaction to this. I'm not exactly fashion-forward where my hair is concerned. Basically, I've had the same short hairstyle since tenth grade.

People like Liberace and Lady Gaga wear wigs, not people like me. That is what I thought until I saw my husband nodding his head when the doctor handed us the fake-hair prescription. In a flash I realized it might be easier for Moe to see his cancer-stricken wife in a sort-of-natural-looking wig than in a scarf or a ball cap, at least occasionally. Maybe it would be nice for me, too. Sometimes it takes a crisis before a person is willing to move outside of his or her comfort zone.

Cancer has exploded my comfort zone, and maybe that's not all bad. Maybe it's time I changed some things up. In that spirit, my girlfriend, Angie, and I visited the wig shop at Virginia G. Piper Cancer Center last week. The woman who waited on us had been through chemo twice and lost her hair both times.

"Will I lose my eyebrows and lashes?" I asked as she rolled a nylon stocking down my skull to flatten my still-intact locks.

"I didn't," she said.

Over the next 45 minutes, I discovered that anything red, reddish, grayish or platinum does not belong on my head. Big hair doesn't work, either. Ix-nay on the Tina Turner. A few times, I was buried under so much hair I looked like one of those poodles whose fur has overgrown its face. "I don't think so," Angie would say politely, a slight frown on her face. Translation, "Hideous!"

Finally, we settled on a short "frosti blonde" wig that might actually be an improvement over my own boring brown hair. You can form your own opinions when you see me wearing it in a few weeks … if I can muster the courage.

Postscript: Though I fully intended to "rock that wig," it never happened. At first it was because chemo had made my scalp too tender to tolerate a hairpiece. Weeks later, when the pain was gone, I gave it another try. No matter how I adjusted the wig, the image in the mirror didn't look like me. I hated that false image—so much that it made me cry. Breast cancer may have stolen my hair temporarily, but I could not let it steal my identity. Instead of a wig, I covered my head in hats, scarves, or nothing at all. While it was hard for my family to see me that way, they understood and accepted my decision. "A wig would not have made you look more like your old self," my husband said recently.

The Letter

Thursday, September 15, 2011

The morning before my first chemotherapy infusion, my seventeen-year-old daughter handed me a sheet of paper folded in thirds. "Read this after I leave for school," she said. I unfolded it as soon as she went out the door.

> Dear Mom,
>
> Today is the big day. It's scary and surreal and weird and nerve-wracking. But it's here. I wish I could be there with you today, but I want you to know that I will be thinking of you all day, along with your hundreds of other supporters. I also want you to know that I believe you are going to make it through this….

I wiped away some tears and read on:

You are healthy, strong, persistent and full of more courage than I will ever know. Which is why I know you're going to be okay…. In my entire life, I have never once seen you give up on a goal…. It's just like you said, this is one more challenge you need to overcome. And you will.

You are my role model, my therapist, my rock, my best friend, and my mom all at the same time. I look up to you more than you could possibly know. I may not say it, but I love spending time with you….

So today, try to remember all the wonderful memories we share…. None of that is going away. In fact, I am anticipating having many more stories to tell, places to see, and things to experience.

You have a fight ahead of you. But it is a fight you can win. You are going to make it through this. And if you ever feel like your strength is wavering, remember all of the people who are rooting for you….

Good luck today. Stay strong, you can do this….

That's not the entire letter, but you get the idea. I don't know what I did to deserve a daughter like Emily. I only know I can't let her down. Tomorrow morning, before I have my second chemo infusion, I will reread her letter. Then I will put on my game face and go take the bitter medicine.

Postscript: Emily's letter is a treasured artifact from my chemo days. More than two years later, a read-through still has the power to lift me up … and to bring tears to my eyes. Emily is in college now, figuring out her particular path to saving the world. Whatever career she chooses, I believe her abilities to communicate and inspire will help her make a positive difference in the lives of many.

Second Chemo

Friday, September 16, 2011

We are doing a few things differently with my nausea meds this time around, and it seems to be working. Eight hours after chemo, I've had no vomiting and only mild nausea. Most likely credit is due to the Sancuso anti-nausea patch that I put on my upper arm 24 hours before chemo, but it could be the diet ginger ale I've been guzzling.

Do I feel good? Well, "good" is a relative term. I feel good compared with last time. I have that overly full feeling in my stomach that you get before a bug takes over. I'm cautiously optimistic that it will pass in the next day or so.

While my stomach is so-so, my spirits are very high. My friend, Pam, who happens to be a nurse, was my guardian angel during chemo this morning. Her presence made the few hours fly by. This evening, I am reading encouraging e-mails and cards, and being spoiled by my husband. I have much to be grateful for.

The Silver Lining

Saturday, September 17, 2011

On receiving my cancer diagnosis, I felt shock, sadness, and fear. One day, I looked out the window into my backyard, dappled in the bright Arizona sunlight. My view stopped at the back wall, and suddenly a shiver went through me. Up until then, I had always thought of my life as extending to the distant horizon, like the view I've had from so many mountaintops. On that day, I realized it might not be so. I could live only a few more years, as far as the back wall so to speak, or another three or four decades.

This wasn't true just for me, now that I had cancer, but for everyone. None of us knows how much time we have. We all know that life is finite, but for most this is an abstract concept until a life-threatening crisis awakens us to our mortality.

My "back wall" moment terrified me. But once I got past the fear, an amazing thing happened. I began to have a greater appreciation for every good thing in my life. The big southwestern sky that I love never looked bluer. The rugged Arizona landscape seemed prettier than ever. A homemade bowl of soup I've made many times brought more intense pleasure to my taste buds. Every kind gesture, message, phone call, and card from a loved one filled me with joy and gratitude.

After "seeing the back wall," I also understood with greater clarity what is most important to me: people, relationships and experiences; honesty, integrity, generosity, and love. If we don't have these, the rest of what we spend our lives striving for will never fill us up.

Next thing you know, I'll be saying "life is groovy," or some other nonsense. Not really. I just wanted to share with you the silver lining of this difficult time in my life. Moe and I are both more "in the moment," finding ways to enjoy and appreciate each day. Yesterday, after my second chemo treatment, we got to work updating our bucket list. Trips to Hawaii and Ireland are at the top, but it's a long list and extends well into the future.

Postscript: Since my wake-up call, we have been working our way through the bucket list and made a priority of being with loved ones. Our most precious commodities are not money, possessions, beauty, brains, sex, or even health. They are love and time.

Random Act of Kindness

Sunday, September 18, 2011

Last week, after I found out my white count was back up, I decided to go shopping for a new recliner. Oh, we have a recliner, a very nice

La-Z-Boy, but it's a rocker-style recliner. Nothing is worse than sitting in a rocker when you are queasy after chemo. Even the seconds it took in the rocker to pull the lever to recline put my stomach over the edge. If I was going to put my feet up, I needed a non-rocking recliner, preferably before my next chemo on Friday.

At 4 p.m. on a Monday, you could have driven monster trucks down the empty aisles of the furniture store. The lone salesman was only too happy to show me his recliners, few of which were non-rocking and none that would work for me. When he offered to order a chair that might suit, I explained to him why I needed a non-rocker, and soon.

All of a sudden his eyes got wide and he exclaimed, "My sister had breast cancer and she had the exact same problem. I want your business, ma'am, but I'm going to show you something."

He led me to one of his rocker/recliners, lifted up the back so I could see the rocking mechanism, and explained how to insert a block of wood into it to prevent the rocking. He was rewarded with a big smile, many thanks, and a promise that he would get my business at some time in the future.

That evening, I told my handy husband how to neutralize the rocker, and he got the job done before my next chemo. The chair still rocks a little, but not enough to make me feel sick. I may yet buy a stationary recliner, but thanks to a kind-hearted furniture salesman I no longer have to be in a hurry about it.

"Do What You Feel Like Doing"

Monday, September 19, 2011

A couple of times, I've asked my oncologist whether I should restrict my active lifestyle during chemo. He always gives the same answer: "You can do what you feel like doing." I love that attitude.

He knows very well that the nausea and fatigue that accompany chemotherapy will set limits for his patients. But he's not going to. The overall message from my doctor and his staff is to keep living your life as much as possible during treatment.

I've taken them at their word. Two days after my first chemo, I started walking in the park. Six days later, I hiked to a familiar mountaintop. The weather was hot, and I had to rest a few times, but I made it. The next week, in cooler weather, I tackled two more local mountaintops. One of them was Camelback Mountain, the day before my second chemo. And yes, I needed a nap afterward.

I didn't go alone, and probably wouldn't have attempted these hikes at all, except for the support of my "OEBs," Pam, Angie and Barclay. (Obsessive Exercise Buddies, in case you were wondering.) In normal times, we OEBs hike or bike together three times a week. Though I am slower than usual, these strong women are still hiking and walking with me, and teaching me about true friendship.

I'm going to keep hiking up mountains for as long as I can because it is powerful medicine for me. I'm also going to blog, see friends, and follow the usual routines at home as much as I am able. Life is not all gloom and doom when you're fighting cancer. In fact, sometimes it's very good.

Goodbye, Hair

Tuesday, September 20, 2011

I knew I was going to lose my hair, but nothing prepared me for the cascade of loose locks that poured over my body in the shower after my second chemo treatment. Or for the fist-size clumps of brown that filled my brush each time I ran it across my head. Finally, I said, "Enough!" and made an appointment with my hairdresser.

If I had to watch my hair go away, quick and painless seemed better than slow and agonizing. So, today at 11 a.m., I went to see Iva, our family hairstylist and friend who has been cutting Moe's hair since his medical residency. At my insistence, she got out her clippers and gave me a close buzz cut. Some might say I now look like a Marine recruit, but I prefer to think my new look is more reminiscent of Sinead O'Connor in her heyday.

My good pals Pam and Angie were with me at the hair salon, and even brought wigs to put on so I wouldn't feel strange in mine. Standing between Angie in her Marilyn Monroe and Pam in a blue Avatar do, how could I be sad?

We had just finished taking pictures when Moe showed up. He hid it well, but I could tell he was shocked by my appearance. It got easier for him when I put on a ball cap with hair attached. Maybe it will be better still when my scalp is not so tender and I can tolerate the "frosti blonde" wig. Meanwhile, I'll be donning scarves and hats and reminding myself that this is just another step forward in my quest to overcome breast cancer.

Postscript: Friends insisted I looked "cute" or "cool" without hair. Whether true or not, their approval helped me feel less self-conscious about joining the ranks of Sinead, The Rock, Howie Mandel, and other cue balls. No one ever pointed at my hairless head in horror, though a number of strangers did come up and ask to hug me. Ordinarily, this would have made me uncomfortable, but during chemo I never turned down an unsolicited hug. It always made me feel better, and without the sting of a shot or the side effects of a cancer drug.

Dense Breasts, Not Genes the Likely Culprit

Wednesday, September 21, 2011

After the biopsy that discovered my breast cancer and the MRI that told us it was worse than we first believed, I have been gun shy of test results. Today, however, I got a result that was actually in my favor. The genetic test to determine whether I had the BRCA1 or BRCA2 gene was negative.

This means my breast cancer probably is not linked to the strong family history of prostate cancer on my father's side of the family. It also means I am not at high risk of developing cancer in my other breast or in my ovaries. More importantly, it puts my daughter in a lower risk category where cancer is concerned. Yes, she will have a 1.5 to 2 times greater-than-average risk of getting breast cancer because her mother had the disease. She will *not* have to worry about the 10 to 32 times greater risk associated with BRCA1 and BRCA2.

As our insurance does not cover genetic testing, Moe and I had to pay more than $3,000 out of pocket for this piece of information. After the sticker shock, we agreed that it was money well spent.

So why did I get breast cancer? We might have an answer. While we were waiting for the results of my genetic test, *The New England Journal of Medicine* published a new study on breast cancer screening. It indicated that a woman with dense breasts like mine (most middle-aged women have fatty breast tissue) has a 5 times greater-than-average risk of developing breast cancer. I had no idea, but dense breasts were by far my biggest risk factor for this disease.

Mammograms often are unable to detect cancer in dense, fibrous breast tissue. To other women with dense breasts, I advise the following: If something seems suspicious, have it checked out right away. It may save your life. I hope it saves mine!

Postscript: In 2011, when I was tested for BRCA1 and BRCA2, Myriad Genetics claimed to own the patents for these genes and had a monopoly over testing. Breast cancer patients with a suspicious family history whose insurance didn't cover genetic testing (many insurers, including mine, did not) often didn't get tested. Many could not afford Myriad's $3,000 fee. Since joining the breast cancer sisterhood, I have met several such women.

In 2013, the Supreme Court ruled that a company such as Myriad cannot "own" natural genes, a decision that should end Myriad's lock hold on BRCA1 and BRCA2 testing and make it more affordable. I certainly hope that is the case. Breast cancer patients for whom this testing has been recommended should not have to forego it because of the exorbitant cost. It was a tremendous relief to know that I did not have either BRCA gene mutation and would not be passing them on to my daughter. Only 2 percent of all breast cancer cases involve BRCA1 and BRCA2, but not knowing and worrying would have been awful.

If I'd tested positive, I might have elected to remove not only my cancerous breast, but also my healthy breast and ovaries to prevent future cancers. Some might call that an extreme reaction (and a few did when Angelina Jolie removed her healthy breasts because of her unusually high cancer risk), but it doesn't seem so radical to those of us who have endured a serious bout of cancer or watched a loved one perish from the disease.

Food from the Heart

Thursday, September 22, 2011

In the past, I have made meals for friends whose families were in crisis. Usually, it was when someone was seriously ill, having surgery, or when a family lost a loved one. I didn't do it on my own, but as part of a meal-delivery brigade organized by friends of the stricken family. Never did I imagine that I would one day be the recipient of such support.

Well, that day has come. Since my first chemo infusion on September 2, friends have been bringing dinners to our home on three different nights during the week after each treatment. These have been healthy, delicious repasts plentiful enough to feed my family of four for a few days. I have no doubt that Moe, Brian, and Emily would be woeful and gaunt if not for the sustenance provided by these generous and talented cooks. If you think I'm joking, you don't know about the Bell metabolism!

Though I am often able to walk in the mornings, my energy is flagging by late afternoon, especially during the week after chemo. I am exhausted just by the idea of planning a meal, shopping, and cooking. I'm also supposed to avoid crowded places like the supermarket. Because of the meal brigade, I don't have to worry about it. This is an invaluable gift, and another example of how the support of your community can help you heal.

Thank you Stacy, Barclay, Molly, Penny, Erin, Pam, Sue, and all of the rest of you who have signed up to feed the Bells during our time of need. You ladies are providing so much more than nourishment. When I am once again well and cancer-free, it will be partly because of you.

Quarantine!

Friday, September 23, 2011

Though the week after chemo is not exactly fun for me, this time I think it was worse for my daughter. Emily is a high school senior with a busy social life and a demanding academic load. Like seventeen-year-olds everywhere, she often short-changes herself on sleep to get everything done. She also spends five days a week in the germ incubator that is high school.

On Tuesday—surprise, surprise—Emily came home sick. She had a fever, sore throat, cough, the chills, and chest congestion. This was Moe's worst nightmare: post-chemo wife with dropping white cell count that makes her vulnerable to infection and a sick teenager in the same home. Yikes!

Fortunately, we have a big house. Moe quarantined Emily upstairs and me downstairs. He then bought enough hand sanitizer and antibacterial wipes to inflate stock prices in certain publicly traded companies. Poor Emily spent the next few days upstairs by herself. She was banned from the kitchen and only passed through it briefly, without touching anything, the few times she dragged herself to school.

Moe left food for Emily at the top of the stairs in the morning and carried down her dirty dishes when he got home from work. Harry Potter had it better in the cupboard under the stairs. I told Em I felt like the world's worst mother, but she said, "It's okay Mom, I'll never forgive myself if I get you sick."

As of today, despite a low white cell count confirmed at the doctor's office, I am still well and Emily is on the mend. I got another shot in the arm that should boost my count over the next few days. If I do come down with a fever or chills, my doctor has instructed me to start antibiotics immediately because it could turn into a "very serious situation."

Though I am trying to lead a somewhat normal life, the truth is that chemo makes you vulnerable. The week after an infusion, I should avoid crowds, skip fresh vegetables unless I wash them carefully myself, stay away from anyone who is sick, and wash my hands frequently. If Emily, Brian, or Moe gets sick, quarantine will be imposed.

I hate my vulnerability and how it affects my family, but a card I received in the mail today put things in perspective. "Chemo sucks," it said on its front. Then, inside, "But if it sucks the cancer right out of you, then 'yay chemo!' "

Postscript: My daughter remembers well that day she came home sick. "One of the worst days of my life," she says. That's because it was also the day I had my hair shaved off. Emily was lying on a couch upstairs, feeling ill and worried she'd pass her virus to me, when I came into the doorway to show her my shorn head. I remember the brave face she put on and her encouraging words. Only recently, she admitted that she started crying as soon as I descended the stairs. With my hair gone, she couldn't look at me without being reminded of my cancer.

Brian Comes of Age

Saturday, September 24, 2011

On September 1, the day before my first chemo, my son Brian celebrated his twenty-first birthday. I had been scheduled to start chemo the day before his birthday and was pretty upset when treatment was postponed. In retrospect, it turned out for the best.

In the distant future, when Brian reflects on his life, I hope his recollection of this birthday puts a smile on his face. His dad and I made an extra effort to gather special presents for him, one of which was a six-pack of imported beers recommended by the beer connoisseur who led our family on a brewery tour in Bruges, Belgium in July. This surprise was a big hit.

The best part of the day was the family meal we shared that evening. Moe had made a reservation at a mountaintop restaurant overlooking Phoenix. The four of us sat at a table by the window, from which we watched the sunset over the Phoenix Mountains Preserve and the sprawling city below. We toasted Brian's coming of age, enjoyed gourmet food, and reminisced about our son's life so far.

Never was our family more in need of a celebration. Emily forgot about the tests she had at school the next day, Moe didn't think about work or worry about me, and I tried to put aside the anxiety I felt prior to starting chemo. We were all just there on the mountaintop savoring the experience. Brian seemed truly happy.

People have asked how my children are coping with my cancer diagnosis. As far as I can tell, they are upset by it but dealing pretty well. I have to admit, though, that it is far easier for me to read Emily's emotions than her brother's. Like many young men, my son is not one to talk about his feelings. He hasn't shared with me what it's like to find out your mother has cancer. Or to see her sick after chemo or with her hair shaved off. I can only imagine.

When he feels overwhelmed by what is going on with me, I hope Brian will be comforted by the memory of his family together and celebrating him at the first supper of his adulthood. His mother treasures that memory. My desire to celebrate more special events with my family is a huge incentive to triumph over cancer. If you're reading this Brian, know that I will gladly endure every unpleasant aspect of my treatment to spend more birthdays with you.

Postscript: When Brian turned twenty-one, he had been "taking a break" from college for almost a year. My son was unemployed, living at home, and lacking direction. His dad and I couldn't seem to find the right words or actions to help him move forward. For the next several months, our concerns about Brian's future took a backseat to my health problem. Unbeknownst to us, while I was going through chemo Brian was getting his act together.

The week of my mastectomy, he came out of his bedroom and announced he was going out to get a job. Moe and I stared at him in disbelief, but he was busing tables in a restaurant by the end of the week. A few months later, he was back in school pursuing a math major. It's been full steam ahead ever since. At the moment he is working two jobs and acing every class at Arizona State University. There may be no connection between my cancer battle and Brian's struggle to turn his life around, but to me the two will always seem somehow intertwined. And yes, I'm really proud of him.

True Love

Sunday, September 25, 2011

In one of my favorite movies of all time, *The Princess Bride*, the young farm boy Westley falls hopelessly in love with the fair maiden Buttercup. To win her heart, Westley answers Buttercup's every request, even the unreasonable ones, with the phrase, "As you wish."

For the past several weeks, since we found out about my little problem, my practical, alpha male husband has been treating me like Westley treated Buttercup. I have tried not to abuse my newfound power over Moe, but it hasn't been easy.

He has brought me a dozen red roses four or five times, to the point where I have grown accustomed to fresh-cut flowers in the house. When I said it would make me happy if we bought our daughter a car, he started calling dealerships and we had a new vehicle in the driveway the next weekend. When I asked whether we could temporarily relocate his beloved recliner chair from our bedroom to the family room so I could put my feet up after chemo, he moved it right away. Just the other day, he bought me my own non-rocking recliner.

When I complained about the leaves that had piled up on the rocks in our desert-landscaped front yard, leaves that I would normally rake but that Moe doesn't want me raking right now, he hired two guys with blowers who were working on a lawn up the street to blow all the leaves off of our front yard. This had never happened before.

Moe hates blowers. When he led me out to look at our pristine rock lawn, I beamed my biggest smile at him and said, "This is true love."

I meant it. Moe wasn't bothered about those leaves; he was only concerned with pleasing me. I think he understood that when you have a disease that is out of your control and your life is filled with uncertainty, a little thing like a tidy front yard brings you peace. I don't know how much longer Moe will go on being my genie, but I sure am enjoying the magic carpet ride.

Postscript: My spell over Moe has worn off some since cancer treatment ended. I take that as a sign that he is once again confident in my good health. I will never forget the true love he demonstrated when I was sick, and I know it's still there under the surface of our normalcy.

Good Response

Monday, September 26, 2011

Before I started treatment, I asked my oncologist how long it would be before we could tell whether chemotherapy was working. He told me we might see a noticeable change after just two infusions. Last Friday, the week after my second infusion, the doctor examined the area of my tumor. "It is not easy to find," he said. "This is a good response."

I sat there with my shaved head and itchy, watery chemo eyes and felt waves of joy and hope rush through me. I flashed my husband a quick smile and raised my eyebrows, conveying the message, "This is hard but it's gonna be worth it." He smiled back and nodded.

I wondered whether the doctor had any idea of the power of his words. He is a smart fellow and probably did. Even though his conclusions were not exactly scientific, he is an expert on chemo and cancer, and I trust him. Next time around, when the going gets tough, the words "good response" will be running through my mind, encouraging me to hang on.

Seeing What Is Possible

Tuesday, September 27, 2011

You know how when a new model of car catches your eye and afterward you start seeing that car all over the road? Well, when you get breast cancer, it's that way too. All of a sudden, everywhere you turn, there's an article or TV news clip on it, a friend with a friend or relative who had it, an ad for a local medical center that specializes in it, a song on the radio about it, a special diet designed to prevent it ... and so on.

I have read lots of articles, heard numerous celebrity recovery tales, and even bought a cookbook to help me fight breast cancer. However, it is the survivors I've encountered that inspire me most.

One of them, Pat, is in my bunko group. A dedicated and respected elementary school teacher, Pat has spent decades helping her students cultivate a love of learning. She taught at my children's school but was not one of their teachers. Still, I remember when she was diagnosed. She had surgery and chemotherapy and kept right on teaching as many days as she could.

Pat was never defined by her disease. Within a short time, she stopped being thought of as the teacher who had breast cancer and was once again Pat K., one of the best educators at our school.

A few weeks ago, when I dropped in at bunko for a few hours, Pat welcomed me with a big hug. "This year I celebrate thirteen years cancer-free," she said, her warm eyes sparkling. "I have been where you are, and you will get through it." I looked at this vibrant, confident woman, and felt hope. Her very presence in the room made me see what is possible for me.

"If there is anything you need, or you want to talk, call me," she added. I will, Pat, but I want you to know that you've helped me a great deal already.

Postscript: Pat continues to be a model of resiliency. She is one of several long-term survivors who have shown me the way forward from breast cancer. They no longer think about the disease every day. The possibility of recurrence, though very real, does not preoccupy their thoughts. They are too busy making the most of their lives to dwell on the worst-case scenario. While I strive for a "no fear" attitude like theirs, I'm not quite there yet. One's mental and emotional recovery from cancer takes time, sometimes more of it than the physical recuperation.

"You're on Chemo, Stupid"

Wednesday, September 28, 2011

I had big ambitions today. I went on a five-mile walk with a friend in the park. Another friend took me out to lunch. In the afternoon, I planned to go shopping. I had three stops in mind but only made it as far as the car. Like the out-of-shape athlete who can't make it a second time around the track, I was done.

With only two days until my next chemo, I felt an urgency to run errands and be out of the house while I still could. But my body didn't care about my brain's desires. The answer was "No! And by the way, you're undergoing chemo, Stupid."

I went back inside and plopped down in a chair at the kitchen table. Before long, my eyelids were drooping and I dragged myself to the bedroom. Such is the way of things during therapy. I accept it, but I don't have to like it. In fact, it makes me even more determined to take my life back. Note to cancer, "You may have knocked me down today, but I *will* kick your butt in the end."

Camelback Mountain High

Thursday, September 29, 2011

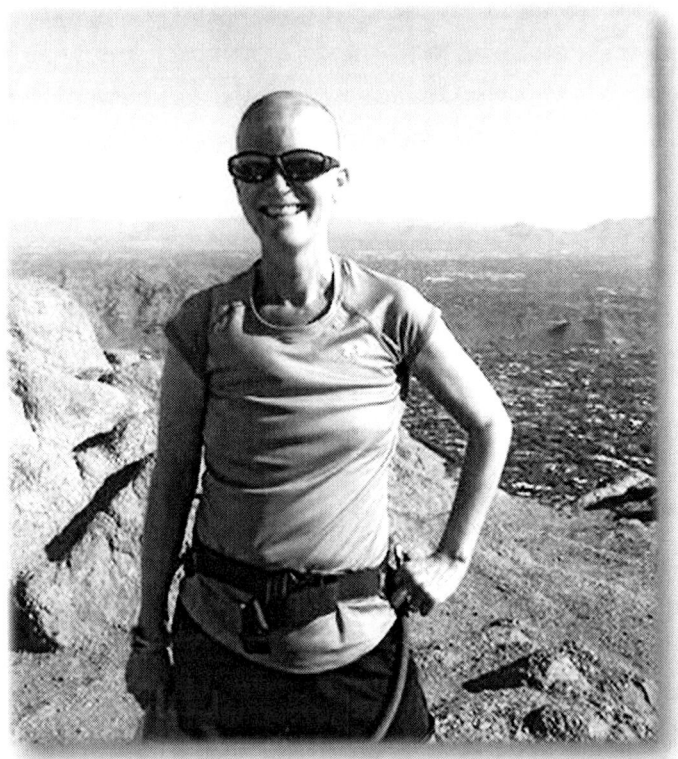

This morning, with some trepidation, I joined my girlfriends for our weekly hike up Camelback Mountain. Last week, I got one mile up the mountain, a quarter-mile from the summit, and had to stop. Still in the first week after chemo, it was all I could do to put one foot in front of the other up the steep, boulder-strewn path. I was pushing to my limits and felt lightheaded.

Today, almost two weeks since my last treatment, I trudged up to the top of the mountain without a hitch. I have been on a "Camelback Mountain high" all day. (See my GI Jane impersonation above.)

Tomorrow, when I go for my third chemo infusion, I will be buoyed by the sweet memory of today.

Postscript: Sometimes I look at photos from my past and don't like what I see. "Too fat," "goofy smile," "stupid pose," "ridiculous clothes"—such is the chatter of my inner critic. When I look at this picture, I have no unkind words. I think, *Who is that crazy woman? I want to be like her.* I can hardly believe that I *am* her. I hiked mountains through chemo. I took my hat off and showed the world my baldness. I did not give up my smile. If I ever have to go through chemo again, I will look to this version of myself to show me the way. She is a warrior, not a victim.

The Canyon Will Be There

Friday, September 30, 2011

The first weekend of October, the past thirteen years in a row, I have gone with friends to hike the Grand Canyon from the South Rim to the North Rim and back. We call it hiking "rim-to-rim-to-rim." We don't do it all at once, but South Rim to North Rim on Saturday and North Rim to South Rim on Monday. Before my diagnosis, I was all set to make the forty-two-mile trek again this year.

Today, instead of getting my third chemo infusion, I should have been driving to the South Rim with my two girlfriends. One of them, Jill, was traveling from Chicago to hike the canyon with me. The other, Angie (my wig advisor), had joined me on this trip the past two years.

We would have packed my trunk full of daypacks, boots, hiking poles, hats, headlamps, trail food, blister remedies, rain jackets, and all the other items on the checklist, then sped away from the hot desert up to cool, piney Flagstaff for a hearty lunch.

Arriving at South Rim Village by late afternoon, we'd have had time to check-in to our motel room and pull on fleece jackets before going to see the sunset over one of the world's great wonders. The view would have wowed me, as it always does. Somewhere along the Rim, we would have encountered other members of the larger group with whom I've been sharing this adventure for the past fourteen years.

Following an early dinner, where calories were no concern, Angie, Jill, and I would have hurried back to the room to get our gear ready. Then, nervous with anticipation, we'd have tried to get some shuteye. Sleep is often fitful when you have a 3:30 a.m. wake-up call and a twenty-one-mile hike ahead of you. I would have told my companions, "Even if you can't sleep, don't worry. Your body is still resting." Those are comforting words when you're still awake at 1 a.m.

I must admit, I'm a little sad to be home this evening recovering from chemo, rather than on the South Rim preparing for my fourteenth canyon crossing. Though I told my girlfriends weeks ago that I couldn't go, I didn't give up my room reservations until early this week. Not a happy moment. Tonight I am reminded of words I have spoken to friends who had to cancel plans to hike rim to rim, "The Canyon will be there when you are ready." I already have my reservations for next year.

Postscript: You'll have to keep reading to find out whether I was able to do the rim-to-rim-to-rim hike in 2012. No skipping ahead.

My Cup Runneth Over

Saturday, October 1, 2011

Yesterday, when I arrived at my oncologist's office for chemo, the receptionist said, "Oh, we have a surprise for you."

Chemotherapy

She presented me with a huge gift bag. The biggest item inside was the softest blanket I have ever felt, velour on one side and faux sheepskin on the other. On a corner of the blanket the word "Courage" was embroidered over a pink ribbon. The bag also contained a white ball cap with the same "Courage" logo, a pink "Walk the Walk" T-shirt, anti-nausea lollipops, lotion, socks, and a journal. I wasn't expecting Christmas at chemo, but there it was.

This was the second time four nurses from Moe's office, Connie, Karen, Judy, and Kathy, have had gifts waiting for me on a chemo day. This time Darleen from billing also joined in. I have known most of these ladies for years. They have given shots to my children and me, taken our vital signs dozens of times, and become good friends. I was not surprised by their generosity, but I was touched.

The Christmas-on-chemo-day theme persisted when I got home and another friend texted me, asking if she could stop by for a few minutes. Laura, a caregiver and friend to my mother-in-law before Fridl passed away, knows a little something about chemo. Two years ago, she was diagnosed with leukemia and had to undergo a stem cell transplant. She spent months in the hospital, enduring a harsh course of chemotherapy designed to wipe out her own faltering bone marrow in preparation for the transplant. Though Laura faced a much greater challenge than mine and had numerous setbacks, her faith never wavered and she regained her health.

Since my diagnosis, Laura has been in close contact with me, sending words of inspiration and encouragement. Yesterday, she dropped by with a loaf of Challah bread and a decorated box full of wrapped items. "This is a Sunshine Box," she explained. "You get to open one present every day."

Wow, I was as giddy as a little kid. The Sunshine Box was like the twelve days of Christmas. I got one surprise yesterday (book), another one today (magazine), and there are several more for the days to come. Chemo day is hard, and all of these ladies know it. Some other days are difficult, too, but not like Day One. Thank you all for your efforts to cheer me up. My cup runneth over.

Postscript: When you get cancer, it brings out the best in your friends and loved ones. Other survivors agree with me on this. My friends rose up like an army to support me through treatment. They blew me away with their kindness. I'm not talking about just my closest buds but also the wider circle of friends I have made over the years but don't see often. My relatives, close and distant, stepped up in a big way as well. Until breast cancer, I never realized how much support was there for me if I needed it. This was a gift of my disease and made me feel blessed.

Nurse Pam

Sunday, October 2, 2011

Yesterday, one day after my third chemo, I went to Virginia G. Piper Cancer Center to receive the Neulasta shot that stimulates my bone marrow. While the shot is painful, I no longer dread it. And it's all because of Nurse Pam.

The first time I received this shot, four weeks ago, I had been vomiting all day following my first treatment and appeared haggard, to say the least. My pale, stressed-out husband didn't look much better. Nurse Pam immediately saw our distress and handled us with utmost care. She explained that Neulasta can cause bone pain, but that many patients have found relief taking Claritin (an over-the counter antihistamine, go figure) and Advil. Pam comforted us with her kind words, and she was right about the Claritin, too.

Two weeks later, when we returned for my second Neulasta shot, Nurse Pam remembered us. "You guys look so much better!"

she said. We were doing better, and it was nice that someone noticed. I started to feel like I would come to the center as much for a dose of Pam as for my shot. On our way out, I remarked to Moe, "It's great to see someone in a job that is so perfectly suited to her personality."

Yesterday, I was only too happy to visit Nurse Pam again. When she finished with my shot, I thanked her for being a ray of sunshine in my chemo process. Since my next infusion will be on a Tuesday, I will get the follow-up Neulasta shot at my doctor's office on Wednesday instead of from Nurse Pam, who only works Saturdays at the cancer center. I don't know when I'll see her again, but one thing's for sure, I won't forget her.

Coincidently, my good friend Pam, who has accompanied me to my second and third chemo infusions, is also a nurse. From my experience, I can only conclude that if your nurse is named "Pam," you'll be in good hands.

Postscript: As a cancer patient, I found that the attitudes and sensitivity of my health care providers affected my treatment experience and my mood dramatically. A kind greeting, a smile, a gentle touch when hooking up a line or giving a shot, the ability to read in one glance how a patient is doing, and knowing what to say or do to make the situation better—for me, these were the traits that made a caregiver beloved. Cancer health care providers, take notice—you make more of a difference than you may ever know.

Third Chemo

Monday, October 3, 2011

This is Day Four of my third chemo cycle. I am done with the anti-nausea drugs, have ripped the Sancuso patch off my upper arm, and my stomach is transitioning back to normal (though this will take a few more days). Three infusions down, five to go.

Third chemo was much like the second. Friday, I was filled to the brim with cancer-killing drugs and anti-nausea meds. I tasted them in my mouth and felt them upsetting my stomach, but did not throw up, thank God. Similar to a pregnant woman enduring intense morning sickness, I needed several small snacks during the day and evening to help stave off nausea. I also felt fatigue, which sometimes made it difficult to concentrate, but was easy to manage compared with the stomach issues. I would gladly take twenty stinging Neulasta and Neupogen shots in place of one more bout of nausea, but alas, that trade is not available.

The important thing is that each day since Friday, I have felt a bit better. The light is bright at the end of the tunnel, and I'm about to move into some better days. Some people don't have any "good" days during chemo. When I start to feel sorry for myself, I think about just how lucky I am to have good days and so much support during treatment.

Kindness from a Stranger

Tuesday, October 4, 2011

Last Thursday, after hiking up Camelback Mountain, I went over to Whole Foods Market for a quick, healthy lunch. I was wearing a scarf to cover my shaved head, a get-up that, though you'd rather it wouldn't, screams "chemo patient." While I was chatting with the lady who was handing out samples, another woman approached me. "Excuse me," she said. "I just want you to know that I was where you are three years ago."

I looked up at her radiant face surrounded by thick, shoulder-length blonde hair. Then I glanced at the rest of her—a fit, healthy body obviously recovered from the cancer that had invaded it. "Thank you for telling me that. It really helps," I said.

She nodded, as if she knew. Perhaps someone had done her the same favor when she was sick, I thought, and now she was passing it on to me. Someday not too far in the future, when my hair has grown back, my turn will come.

You Know You're Having a Good Day when ...

Wednesday, October 5, 2011

1. You get a mile up Piestewa (formerly known as "Squaw") Peak five days after chemo. It may not be the top, but there is a bench to sit on and a beautiful view stretching out before you.

2. A friend you made in ninth grade flies out from Chicago to cheer you up as you recover from chemo. When I was fourteen, I met Elaine in freshman English. She soon recruited me to work in her uncle's Chinese restaurant. We became close friends and have remained so, regardless of the time and distance that have separated us since high school.

3. You receive a care package in the mail from a cousin in Indiana who simply wants to help.

4. Your favorite baseball team wins a second home playoff game in convincing fashion, silencing the commentators who predicted the team's demise and putting a big smile on your husband's face. (Go D-Backs!)

5. Your stomach recovers enough from chemo that you can finally enjoy a full meal. :)

Postscript: When life is humming along smoothly, it's easy to take for granted the simple pleasures. During chemo, I promised myself never to do that again. Since then, I try to enjoy what I'm doing and who I'm with in every moment of the day. I don't tune out in the midst of a conversation or lament that a merely good experience was not a great one. It's all great because I am still on this earth, living my life.

Food Fetish

Thursday, October 6, 2011

Like a pregnant woman, I have had cravings while undergoing chemo. During this latest go-round, while my stomach felt like wet cement was moving through, I yearned not for pickles or ice cream but for a savory turkey burger. Admittedly, this is a weird craving. What can I say? You want what you want.

Today at lunchtime, my girlfriend from Chicago insisted on taking me out for a nice meal. "Let's go someplace with a view," she said. I was thinking Chipotle or Paradise Bakery, but they don't have views. Elaine, who has much more imagination than me, had already decided on Elements, a stylish restaurant at Sanctuary Resort, on the side of Camelback Mountain.

I was wearing jeans, peasant blouse and a headscarf. "I'm not really dressed for Elements, Elaine," I told her self-consciously.

"You're fine," she said, and that was that. Before I knew it, we were seated on the restaurant patio, overlooking the resort pool and much of Paradise Valley. It was sunny and about 75 degrees, a perfect day to dine outside in Arizona.

I worried about what to order. Salads and fresh fruits were out because my white count is down. The doctor says I can't trust that fresh items will be washed thoroughly enough to remove germs and bacteria that could compromise my temporarily fragile immune system. I am allowed cooked vegetables or peeled fruit but didn't see those options on the menu. My eyes scanned almost to the bottom of the page before I spotted, to my surprise, "Turkey Burger." Yes!

As it turned out, this was no dried-out fowl patty, but a luscious moist creation that seemed more like turkey meatloaf in burger form. It was topped with a thin layer of cheddar cheese and set within a bun that had the texture and flavor of a soft pretzel. All I had to do to achieve Nirvana was spread on a little ketchup.

If you are rolling your eyes and thinking, "This is a woman with an unsophisticated palate," you might be right. My taste buds *are* ravaged from three rounds of chemo. All I can say is that this was my most satisfying meal in recent memory. And though I cut the burger in half, expecting to have leftovers, only crumbs remained on my plate by meal's end. Thanks Elaine! I have been losing ground in the weight department, but not today.

Postscript: I haven't been back to Elements since that lunch date. It's not that I don't like the restaurant, just that I want to preserve the memory of my favorite meal during chemo.

Before starting treatment, I asked my doctor whether I should expect to lose weight. He said most women undergoing breast cancer chemotherapy actually pack on pounds because of the steroids mixed in to combat nausea. Perhaps due to my sensitive stomach, or maybe because I continued to exercise, I lost weight, though not to a dangerous level. Gain or lose, the important thing is to keep up nutrition during chemo—and it helps to satisfy a craving when possible.

Change of Scenery

Saturday, October 8, 2011

Sometimes it's good to get away. From a house where you've recently spent too much time. From a third chemo recovery week that was more challenging than the first and second. From the arid desert climate that exacerbates the dry eyes, dry skin, and dry mouth side effects of chemotherapy.

Tonight, we are breathing the moist sea air of San Diego. Moe and I can look out the window of our little condo above the Mission Beach boardwalk and see the waves breaking against the sand. We hear the hypnotic sound of water rushing in and out. We feel all the tension leaving our bodies.

For almost 30 years, we have been regular visitors to Mission Beach. We had already reserved this condo before I was diagnosed with cancer. No crowds and great weather make October a perfect time to be at the beach in San Diego. The first time we met with my oncologist, Moe asked whether this trip was still a possibility. To our delight, the doctor said, "Yes."

So here we are, feeling as though we have used our "Get Out of Jail Free" card. I have never been happier to be in San Diego.

Friend Medicine

Monday, October 10, 2011

A month ago, my friend Elaine (my lunch companion in "Food Fetish") called from her Illinois home to ask how she could help me. "Maybe I could just come out and hold your hand while you are going through chemo," she suggested.

Last Wednesday, five days after my third chemo, Elaine arrived like Mary Poppins flying in with a spoonful of sugar. She helped out around the house, walked with me in the park, bought fabric and made me extra scarves on my old sewing machine, and taught me to knit. She also befriended every member of the family. There is no prescription for a medication called "Elaine," but there should be. After three days with her, we all felt better.

Chemotherapy

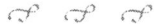

On Saturday, a few hours after Moe and I arrived in San Diego, friends of ours from Orange County drove down to spend the night. Rob and Julie have been part of our lives as long as we have been together. Rob and Moe were best friends in college. When he and Julie got married in 1981, Rob asked Moe to be his best man. Rob returned the favor when Moe and I married in 1983. Since then, we have shared many adventures, camping, hiking, rafting, and backpacking in wild places across the western U.S.

We last saw Rob and Julie at their older son's wedding in June, when we were dressed up and looking our best. When they found out about my diagnosis, Rob and Julie had photos of Moe and me taken by the wedding photographer sent to our home. The man in those pictures looks the same, but the woman has a full head of hair and a few extra pounds. One of the photos is now in a frame on the dresser in our bedroom. I look at it often, as our friends must have known I would, and hope to look like that woman again. In fact, I'm very motivated to make it happen.

Rob and Julie did not arrive in San Diego empty-handed. They brought silk scarves and a bright pink hat for me, and a stack of classic Western novels for Moe. Their greatest gift, of course, was just showing up to spend time with us. Like Elaine, they brought medicine whose value was beyond measure.

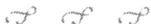

Today at lunchtime, another old pal came to our condo by the beach. Judy and I met during our first year of college in 1977. Though she left after a year to continue her education in Israel, Judy and I kept in touch. Several years ago, she and her family landed in San

Diego, and I have seen her regularly ever since. Our children are close in age, we are both aspiring novelists, and we have both been married to the same guys since 1983. More than that, the intangible something that drew us together when we were eighteen still connects us at age fifty-two. She too arrived here with gifts, an open heart, and a desire to listen and help.

Friend medicine, there's nothing like it.

Postscript: The photo of Moe and me from the wedding we attended two months before my diagnosis still resides on our dresser. A full year went by before my wish came true and I once again looked like the woman in the picture.

Another Mountain High

Tuesday, October 11, 2011

Greetings from San Diego. We are having gorgeous sunny weather at the beach, except for early fog the past two days. This morning, with the coastline enveloped in a cloud, I told my genie I wanted to go for a hike. Specifically, I wished for an uphill trail that would give me a good workout and an inland location where the sun was already shining.

Genie knew I was pining for Camelback Mountain in Phoenix, now that I am feeling better. He understood that my philosophy is to "get while the getting is good" because chemo can rob the strength of mortals the way kryptonite zaps Superman. Clever genie did a little research on the Internet and came up with a Camelback substitute, 1,592-foot Cowles Mountain, the highest point in the city of San Diego.

The 1.5-mile trail up Cowles was not quite as strenuous as Camelback, but it had many of the same features—crowded parking lot, elevation gain near 1,000 feet, and lots of healthy people and their dogs scaling its slopes. After all these years visiting San Diego, I don't know how we missed this gem of a hike. But that was before my husband turned into a genie catering to my every whim, which probably explains it.

A twenty-minute drive from the flat terrain of the beach brought us to the rolling scrublands of Mission Trails Regional Park and the trailhead for Cowles Mountain. On the way up the peak, among the usual hiker types we encountered twenty-some Buddhist monks, indicating that this must be a good and spiritual place. It felt that way to me, too.

Years ago, I wrote an article called, "High Points of San Diego." I visited Mount Soledad, the Old Town Presidio, Mount Helix, Point Loma, and a few other places. None of them had the mojo or matched the 360-degree panorama you get from atop Cowles Mountain. Especially at this time in my life, just being there felt like a gift. Thank you, genie.

Postscript: Moe and I revisited Cowles Mountain recently. The view from the top was just as stunning as the first time, while the hike seemed a little easier. For me this peak is not only a geographical high point, but also a landmark of my cancer journey. It reminds me of how far I've come since then.

Rare Bird

Friday, October 14, 2011

I like to hike up mountains; my husband likes to hike, bike, and chase down birds. Thursday morning, it was his turn, and he took me on a wild goose chase. We drove northeast from the beach to Scripps Ranch Lake in search of the elusive cackling goose. Moe spotted our bird in less than ten minutes and beckoned me to look through his spotting scope. What I saw was a dead ringer for a Canada goose only a lot smaller, about the size of a mallard.

Though I do not keep a bird list like Moe, who has spotted more than 500 North American species, I appreciate the beauty and diversity of our planet's avian life. I especially like the places we go in search of this bird or that. From Scripps Ranch, we headed northwest to Encinitas, on the hunt for an American redstart. We tromped around a small park across the street from the town library, checking every tree and bush. Moe identified warblers, bushtits, phoebes, doves, and mockingbirds, but no American redstarts. Oh well, one out of two isn't bad.

Today, Moe and I went to see *The Big Year,* a movie based on a true story about a select group of obsessive birders who compete to spot the most bird species in a calendar year. The winner counted an amazing 755 species. Moe and I loved this film. He had actually been to some of the places in the movie, and I could relate to the lonely spouses the birders left behind.

It was the perfect end to our week in San Diego, and a nice prelude to Moe's birthday tomorrow. I am grateful to have had several good days this week, when he didn't have to worry about me and could enjoy a relaxing vacation following two of the most stressful months of his life. Though I may be the one with breast cancer, Moe and I are a closely hitched team, and my disease is almost as hard on him as it is on me. He hasn't faltered under the extra weight he's had to carry lately, and I have to say, no wife ever had a better teammate. Among husbands, he may be a rare bird.

Doing a Chore

Sunday, October 16, 2011

Before we left for San Diego, just thinking about the next chemo made my stomach churn. Now, a week later, I feel differently. Several good days in a different environment changed my perspective and lightened my mood. I thought my sense of humor might be gone for the duration of chemotherapy, but this weekend I caught myself making jokes and laughing.

My fourth chemo is only two days away, but I am not approaching it with dread. It is simply a chore that must be done. An evil chore, I will grant you. Worse than changing poopy diapers, scrubbing toilets, or trying to remove the bad smell from the garbage disposal. Worse than disciplining an irrational teenager, calming an angry spouse, or catering to an unreasonable boss. Chemo is worse than all of those chores combined, but it's still just a chore. With time, perseverance and patience, you get through it.

I already know that my stomach will not like the fourth chemo, but eventually the bad days will give way to better ones. I will find myself halfway through the chemotherapy process. I will be able to say good-bye to Adriamycin and Cytoxan and the intense nausea they produce. Those will be reasons to cheer. Chemo Nos. 5–8 will feature a different cancer-killing drug called Taxol. It has unpleasant side effects of its own, but is supposed to be easier on the stomach.

At a certain point, you get tired of the same old chore. A different assignment, even if it's still difficult and onerous, starts to sound good. And so you begin again. With time, perseverance and patience, I will adjust to Taxol and I will get through four more chemo infusions. Then, sometime before Christmas if all goes well, my chemo chore will be finished. I can tell you right now that I won't find a better present than that under the Christmas tree this year.

Fourth Chemo

Wednesday, October 19, 2011

Last week my San Diego friend Judy gave me a small box with a note that said, "Don't open until chemo day." I am like a small child who does not like to wait to open presents, but I *did* wait. Yesterday, before going to my fourth chemo treatment, I opened the box. Inside was a small heart-shaped stone of "ocean jasper."

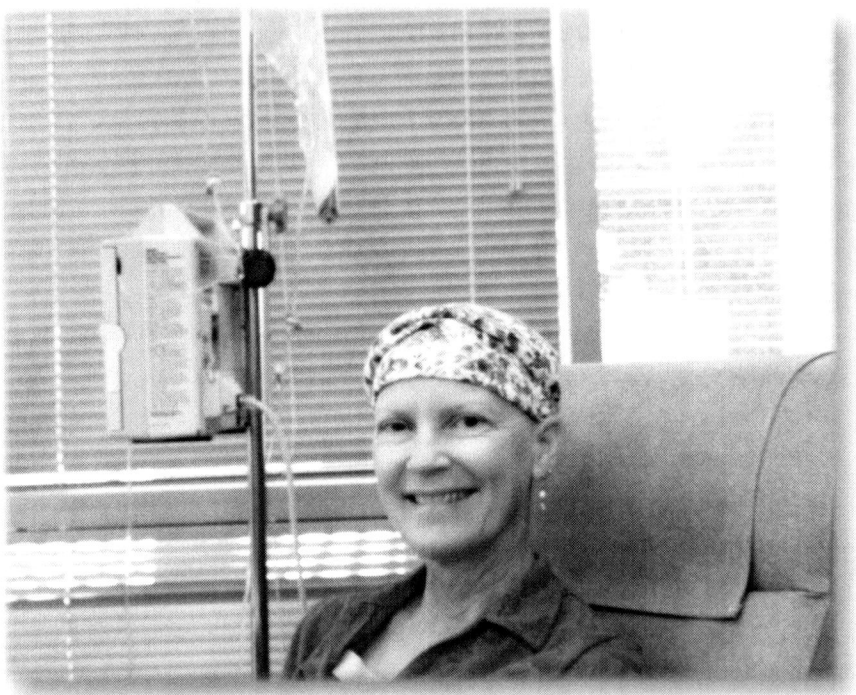

A note that came with the stone described many wonderful properties. To name a few, "It is very healing of the emotions and brings peace of mind…. Ocean jasper is beneficial to digestion, digestive organs, removing toxins…. It is a stone of joy and high spirits…. It banishes complacency and the habit of taking one's loved ones, health, prosperity or security for granted. It brings one's consciousness to the present moment, relieving worry about the future or bitterness about the past." Thank you, Judy. I brought the stone to chemo with me and have kept it nearby ever since.

My friend Barclay drove me to treatment this time. She gave me another gift by teaching me to play Sudoku on my iPad. She assures me that this number game will provide good distraction while I am dealing with the nausea and fatigue that follow chemo. I hope she is right. I need some new distractions. You can only watch so much HGTV and CNN, and it's hard to read a book when you are prone to fall asleep after a page or two. Maybe they have crosswords for the iPad, too.

I felt too crummy to post last night, but am doing much better this morning. Four chemos down, four to go. Though I can't see the finish line, it's nice knowing I'm halfway through the race.

Postscript: Midway through chemo, I felt like the Tortoise in *The Tortoise and the Hare.* "Slow and steady wins the race, slow and steady wins the race..." ran on a continuous loop inside my brain, along with another encouraging line from children's literature, "I think I can, I think I can, I think I can..." from *The Little Engine That Could.*

Disappointment Cleaver

Thursday, October 20, 2011

In 1987, Moe and I decided to get our feet wet in mountaineering by doing a guided climb up Washington State's highest peak, 14,410-foot Mount Rainier. A volcanic mountain topped by glacial ice rutted with crevasses, Rainier demanded more than basic hiking skills.

The guide service required prospective climbers to complete a one-day snow school prior to the two-day summit climb. In snow school, we learned how to put on "crampons," the metal cleats that attach to boots for traction on ice; use an ice axe to stop our fall if we lost footing on a steep slope; securely attach harnesses that would allow us to hook into a rope; and travel on a four-person rope team without getting tangled up.

On a glacier, where crevasses often are hidden under soft layers of snow, the rope might save your life. An unsuspecting climber traveling solo can easily fall through the snow and into one of these fissures and never be seen again. If you're attached to teammates on a rope, however, they will see or feel your fall, use their ice axes to anchor themselves and the rope to the ice, and stop your descent into the crevasse. Then, if you're lucky, you'll get rescued.

While teaching us these new skills, the guides were also assessing each climber's fitness and ability to perform the necessary tasks. It was a strenuous day, but Moe and I were deemed fit enough to begin the 9,000-foot, two-day summit climb the next morning.

Day one of our climb was glorious and exhilarating. Sunny but not overly warm, the conditions were perfect for kicking steps up steep snowfields from Paradise Ranger Station at 5,300 feet to Camp Muir at 10,000 feet. Since we weren't yet on ice, we didn't have to bother with crampons or ropes.

That night, the guides told us to go to sleep right after dinner. Fifteen climbers squeezed into a tiny hut and tried to get some shut-eye. Just after midnight, we arose to prepare for our summit climb and found a blizzard going on outside. The guides delayed for an hour before deciding it would be safe to proceed. Because of the delay, they told us there would be no time to lose. We needed to reach the summit between 8 and 9 a.m. so that we could safely descend before the sun warmed the glacial ice enough to make it slippery and dangerous.

So began one of the most arduous days of my life. Moe and I were put on different rope teams—not a good idea to have spouses on the same team, according to the guides. We set out up the mountain in all our heavy gear, headlamps lighting our way through swirling snowflakes, each of us roped to three strangers.

Our group stopped to rest every hour just long enough to eat and drink, and then pressed on. Within a couple of hours, a few climbers had already dropped out. The guides left them in sleeping bags in sheltered spots along the trail, to be picked up on the way down. The rest of us continued a relentless ascent, as the blizzard cleared and the sky began to lighten. After five hours, we came to a landmark called Disappointment Cleaver. Climbing the precipitous slope from the base of the Cleaver to its top took almost everything I had. I collapsed in a heap on the snow, along with everyone else.

Disappointment Cleaver got its name for a reason. It has turned back many a climber on Mount Rainier. That day, of the fifteen climbers who started for the summit, only six made it past the Cleaver. I'm proud to say Moe and I were among them, and I was the only woman. I remember sitting exhausted on top of the Cleaver and telling myself, "You didn't come all this way to quit just because you feel tired."

An hour-and-a-half later, our diminished group reached the Mount Rainier summit crater and Moe and I saw the sun rising out of a sea of clouds. We felt like we were on top of the world, in more ways than one.

What I learned that day about persevering and enduring through extremely challenging situations has served me well. It is helping me today to stay strong, press on, and do what I must, despite the Disappointment Cleavers in my path, to become cancer free.

Postscript: On our Hawaiian honeymoon in 1983, Moe and I began a quest to stand on the highest point of every state in the U.S. We reached the top of Mauna Kea, on the Big Island, with an assist from astronomers driving to the observatory near the summit. That leisurely beginning high point was a far cry from Mount Rainier, the first of the truly difficult American peaks we tackled.

In 1999, during a three-week expedition, Moe reached the top of Alaska's Mount McKinley (Denali), his fiftieth high point. I stopped at forty-nine (Wyoming's Gannett Peak, 2001), notching every U.S. high point except for Denali. I never dreamed that lessons from our "high-pointing" hobby would one day help me fight cancer, but I'm certain that they did.

Anniversary

Saturday, October 22, 2011

Today Moe and I have been married for twenty-eight years, half of his life and more than half of mine. So many thoughts have run through my mind today, such as, "Why him?" "How did so much time go by?" and "What makes a marriage last?"

There are no pat answers. All I know is that Moe and I each count our wedding day as one of the happiest of our lives. Neither of us experienced cold feet at the time or has since regretted getting married.

We reached our decisions to make a commitment in very different ways, however. Instinct and intuition told me that Moe was "the one," whereas he went through a cerebral process weighing the pros and cons of marriage. His pro-con list was almost a deal breaker for me. Surely feelings should trump practicality when it came to commitment, I thought.

Later, when my annoyance receded and I really thought about it, I realized two things. First, if a marriage between us was going to work, I had to respect his way of making decisions and he had to respect mine. And second, if I was honest with myself, I had already made my own mental pro-con list on the way to deciding he was Mr. Right. ;)

After twenty-eight years, it appears that we were on exactly the same page when it came to commitment. We married for better or worse, for richer or poorer, through sickness and health. I really wish we were not facing the challenge of "sickness," especially on our anniversary. I never expected to be the sick one, but I am thankful to be married to a steady guy who will be there for me and love me no matter what. It's very clear to me that a partnership like ours is one of the best things life has to offer.

Postscript: A life crisis like cancer has the power to bring two people closer together or drive them apart. It will not leave you and your partner unchanged. Moe and I were close before but are closer now. While the possibility of recurrence hangs like a cloud over our future, its presence makes us gentler with each other. The cloud puts petty arguments into perspective. It makes us express the deep feelings couples sometimes leave unspoken. It also makes us judicious about how we spend our time, less of it apart and more together. I won't lie—the cloud causes anxiety, too, but by sharing our worries, Moe and I often are able to let them go.

Out of the Fog

Monday, October 24, 2011

Yesterday, for the first time in five days, my stomach wasn't queasy when I awoke in the morning. That alone made me want to dance a little jig, but it wasn't the only change I noticed. The synapses of my brain, which had been slowed by the chemo drugs, seemed to be firing at their usual speed once again.

"Chemo brain" is a real phenomenon. It makes you forgetful, slower in your thinking, unable to find words, and less capable of multitasking. I believe the effect on me has been fairly subtle so far, but anyone who spoke to me last week might disagree. On Wednesday and Thursday, especially, I had trouble keeping track of phone messages, remembering conversations, and getting out the words that were on the tip of my tongue. I did silly things like put dirty dishes into the dishwasher with clean ones. And yes, it took a lot longer than usual to assemble a coherent blog post.

Even by Saturday, my mind still felt fatigued and a little dull. Though I would have liked to "snap out of it" for our anniversary, I needed two naps and still went to bed by 9:30. Fun girl!

For the average person, waking up to a "normal" brain and a settled stomach is no big deal, but for someone five days out from a chemo infusion, it is a turning point and a victory. The best thing about feeling lousy on Saturday was how much it made me appreciate coming out of the fog on Sunday.

Moe and I went on an easy five-mile hike in the desert, grateful for the warm sun and a cool breeze. We admired the spiky cacti and rugged mountains outlined against the sky, the birds calling from their perches in the green-trunked palo verde trees, and the view of our city spread out before us at our destination overlook. Before I had cancer or ever was affected by chemo brain, I might have taken such an experience for granted. Not anymore.

Postscript: I know chemo robbed me of some brain cells, but I try not to think about it. Am I as sharp as I used to be? Maybe not, but it seems I'm no worse off than any other menopausal fifty-something who can't remember why she went into the next room.

"I Can't Feel a Thing"

Tuesday, October 25, 2011

Today, one week after my fourth chemo, I went for blood tests and a check-up at the oncologist's office. After my second chemo, the soonest we could expect a detectable response, the doctor examined the area of my tumor and said, "It's not easy to find. This is a good response." After the third chemo, he told me the tumor seemed much smaller. This time, he felt the area twice before saying, "I can't feel a thing."

"That's really good, isn't it?" I said.

"Really good," he answered with a smile.

"This makes it all worthwhile," I told him, referring to chemotherapy.

There was other good news, too. First, my white count was the best it's been the week after chemo, so good that I didn't need a Neupogen shot today. Second, my next chemo treatment may be a little easier to bear. Starting next Wednesday, I switch to another chemo drug, Taxol, which tends to have less severe side effects and require less anti-nausea medication than Adriamycin and Cytoxan.

I held my tears until Moe and I got in the car and then let them flow. Chemotherapy is one of the hardest challenges I have ever faced. Like the longest endurance hike, it pushes you to your limits physically and emotionally. Unlike any hike, however, chemotherapy is part of a fight for your life. You can't throw in the towel and say, "I'll try again next year." Not if you want to win the fight, anyway.

Given the high stakes, imagine how it felt to hear the doctor say, "I can't feel a thing." Those words are still ringing in my ears, filling me with joy, relief and hope.

Postscript: Before cancer, few of my friends had ever seen me cry. The disease—along with grinding months of treatment—shattered my ability to camouflage my feelings. It stripped me not only of my hair and the rosy glow of health I'd enjoyed my entire life, but also of my emotional defenses. During treatment, each moment seemed more raw and real than at any previous time in my life. I felt everything on a deeper level, and my emotions were there for all to see.

As I recovered, the intensity of life with cancer subsided, and the mask that hides my most vulnerable self slipped back into place. That mask is not so impervious as before cancer, however. While I am relieved to no longer shed tears at the drop of a hat, I have learned that strong feelings are no cause for shame and should not always be hidden.

Boring Is Beautiful

Wednesday, October 26, 2011

Today I hiked up a mountain (slowly) with my girlfriends, cleaned my kitchen, shopped for groceries and cooked dinner for my family. Tonight I am appreciating the blessing of a normal day. From my cancer-altered perspective, boring is beautiful!

Never Fear, Mom Is Here

Friday, October 28, 2011

At age fifty-two, I am lucky to be able to say that my mother is still alive and well. When I found out about my illness, she was far away in Washington state, where she has spent her summers the past several years. "I haven't been on an airplane in ten years," she said, "but for you I will fly again. If you need me right now, just say the word."

I told her that wouldn't be necessary. I knew she and her boyfriend, Ed, would be driving back to Southern California in October. They could make the five-hour drive to my house in Arizona once they had relocated to their winter home near Palm Springs. I told Mom it would give me something to look forward to.

My mother and I have kept in close contact by phone the past two months. She has kept me laughing with comments such as, "If you were big like Dolly Parton, losing a breast would be a lot more noticeable than it will be on you." So true, and thanks for pointing that out Mom!

More seriously, she has been steadfast in her belief that my cancer will be cured. "You're going to get through this and be just fine, Carrie. There's no way this can come out any other way." When she speaks those words, she makes me a believer, too.

Finally, yesterday, Mom, Ed, and their toy dachshund Willy wheeled into my driveway in their SUV. My house wasn't as clean as usual, I had a scarf on my head instead of hair, and I worried that my mother might be upset at the sight of her daughter with cancer. If she was, she didn't show it. "You look great," she said, wrapping me in a big hug. "I love that scarf."

Last night, Moe and I took Mom to see Emily perform the Napoleon Dynamite dance at her high school's talent show. While we were waiting for Em's act to go on, Mom said to Moe, "Carrie's friends have been really wonderful since she's been sick. They must think a lot of her."

To which my husband replied drily, "Yeah, she's fooled a lot of people."

Mom thought that was the funniest comment she'd heard in decades. Her easy laughter was infectious. I look forward to hearing it all weekend.

"Breaking Bad"

Monday, October 31, 2011

I had an off day yesterday. Oh, it started out well enough. We waved goodbye to Mom, Ed, and Willy, who headed home to Palm Springs after a long weekend with us. Then Moe coaxed me into an outing to Fountain Hills, a town about twenty minutes east of here whose focal point is a manmade lake with a fountain that shoots water 560 feet into the air. It used to be the world's tallest fountain until somebody in the Middle East built a bigger one.

Moe arrived at Fountain Hills seeking an unusual bird someone had spotted in the lake. I just wanted to walk as fast as possible along the path that follows the shoreline. With my next chemo three days away, I was antsy, irritable, and had zero patience for bird watching.

Stupid birds, I thought. *Stupid water jetting skyward. Stupid Superstition Mountains rising like a purple-blue mirage to the east of*

Fountain Hills. Stupid McDowell Mountains to the west, whose high point, Thompson Peak, I have climbed dozens of times. Stupid perfect day.

My husband had seen this mood before and knew that twenty minutes outdoors in a beautiful place would send it packing—that plus three laps around the lake and a short hike up a ridge for a panorama of a prime Sonoran Desert setting. Along the way, we located his target bird and several others newly arrived for the winter season. I stopped grumbling and forgot all about chemo.

Over lunch at a patio table with a view of the lake, we wondered why we don't visit Fountain Hills more often. I apologized to Moe for being such a grump. I try hard to maintain a positive attitude, but I can't do it all the time. Sometimes this stupid cancer thing really gets to me. I am glad for Moe and all the good people in my life who help me back to the light when my mood is breaking bad.

Anticipation

Tuesday, November 1, 2011

It has become my tradition to hike to a mountaintop the day before chemotherapy. This morning I went with my friend Pam to Piestewa Peak, a rugged high point in the Phoenix Mountains Preserve. Last week I made it two-thirds of the way up before exhaustion forced me to stop. I waited at a bench with a view while my companions continued the climb.

Today, two weeks out from my last chemo, I strode past that bench to the top of the peak. The rocky stair steps to the summit seemed to go on and on. I was winded and tired, the way I sometimes feel on a 14,000-foot peak in Colorado. As I used to tell my children during hikes when they were small, "Slow and steady wins the race." I *did* feel like a winner standing on top of the mountain.

That small achievement helped relieve some of my apprehension about tomorrow and how my body will react to the new chemo drug,

Taxol. The infusion will take around four hours, nearly twice as long as previous chemos, and I will be mildly sedated with Benadryl. Taxol side effects include tingling in the fingers and toes, body aches, and mild nausea. Nothing I can't handle, I keep telling myself, but like the night before a journey into unknown territory, there is an element of uncertainty.

No matter. I hiked up a mountain today and I am weary. Neither wild horses nor worries about tomorrow will keep me from a good night's sleep.

Fifth Chemo

Wednesday, November 2, 2011

I am sitting in the chemotherapy suite at my doctor's office, waiting for lab results that will tell us whether to proceed with treatment. This time, I have a reclining chair by the window and can see the McDowell Mountains where I often hike.

When I arrived here this morning, another gift bag was waiting for me. Inside I found a beautiful crocheted prayer shawl, peppermint lip balm, lavender-scented lotion with shea butter, and CDs on "Self-Healing with Energy Medicine" by Dr. Andrew Weil. This is the third time the nurses from Moe's office have showered me with gifts. Thank you again, Connie, Kathy and Karen. You have no idea how much you have cheered me up on chemotherapy days.

I am not alone in the chemo suite. It's a big room full of recliners and most of them are full. The chairs are too far apart for me to chat comfortably with other patients, but I know they are getting chemo for a variety of cancers. All of us are hooked up to IV poles holding bags of cancer-killing fluids.

Shortly after my labs came back, indicating today's chemo was a "go," the nurse hung a bag of Benadryl (to prevent an allergic reaction to the Taxol) on my pole. Within minutes, I couldn't keep my eyes open. Now, an hour-and-a-half later, a half-empty bag of Taxol is dripping through a tube into the port in my chest. I am coming out of the haze of Benadryl and thinking about lunch. So far, so good.

Post-chemo

Thursday, November 3, 2011

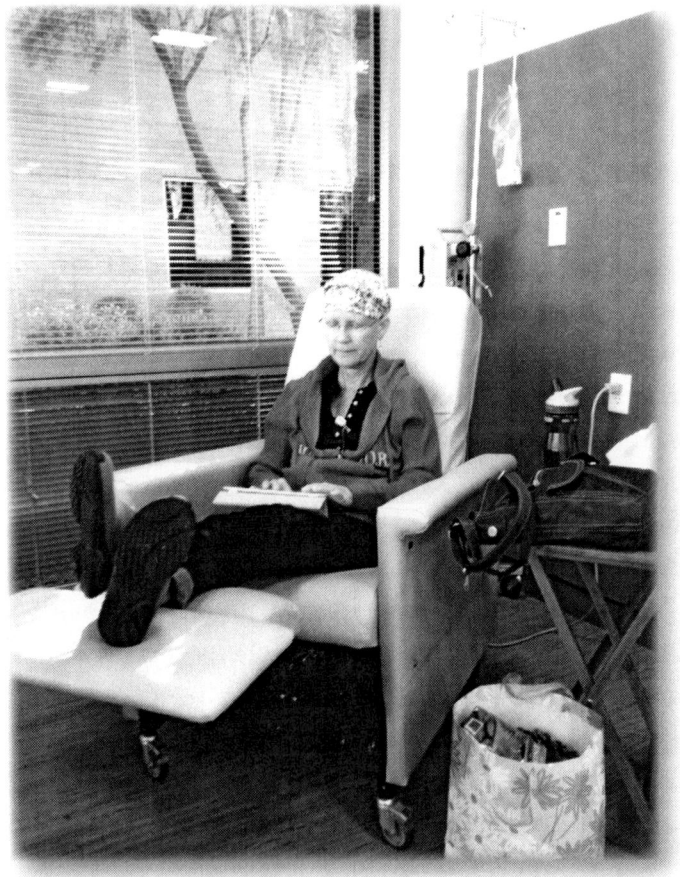

Above: Moe took this photo while I blogged during chemo yesterday.

One day after my fifth chemo infusion, I awoke full of energy, planning to take a walk after breakfast. Somehow, it never happened. By 9 a.m. I was tired. Not sleepy, just not up to a walk. I spent the morning nestled in my recliner with a good book, barely rousing myself by 1 p.m. to go to the doctor's office for my Neulasta shot.

Taxol is far less nauseating than Adriamycin and Cytoxan. Thank God! I will take fatigue over nausea any day. Tomorrow, tired or not, I will be dragging myself out to the park for a walk. Tempting as it might be, you can't keep up your strength lounging in the recliner all day.

No Pain, No Gain

Saturday, November 5, 2011

According to a handout my oncologist provided, Taxol's most common side effect is pain in the joints and muscles, occurring two to three days after receiving the drug. I knew about this effect before my recent infusion, but now I can say I've experienced it firsthand. The pain began yesterday in my hips, thighs, lower back, shoulders, and ankles. I would compare it to the body aches you get with the flu, minus the fever and chills.

The mild to moderate "arthralgias and myalgias" have continued through today and feel the same whether I'm sitting in a chair at home or walking in the park. The handout said the discomfort would resolve in a few days, so I am hoping to be rid of it by tomorrow. Meanwhile, I am getting some relief from Extra Strength Tylenol.

Though the body aches kept me from going with Moe to our cabin, where it is snowy and cold this weekend, I'm grateful to be achy rather than queasy this time around.

The "C" Word

Monday, November 7, 2011

The "C" word I refer to in the heading above is not "cancer." Nor is it "chemo." If you don't want to be grossed out, stop reading right now. At the suggestion of my husband, Moe, a family physician keen on preventive medicine, today's topic is an unsavory aspect of chemo that no one talks about: constipation.

This "C" word made my life miserable for a while yesterday. Without being overly descriptive, let's just say I have never understood the phrase "sh–– a brick" the way I do now. (Sorry, but I did warn you.)

You are probably thinking, "Pff, constipation is no big deal. Everyone deals with it." That may be true, but trust me, chemo drugs and the anti-nausea/anti-allergic-reaction meds that go along with them back up your bowels worse than the most sinful low-fiber diet.

My oncologist had warned me of this. "Chemo slows everything down," he explained prior to my first infusion. "Whatever you do, don't get constipated. Drink plenty of prune juice." At the time I was more worried about throwing up, and rightfully so as it turned out. To prevent vomiting, however, the doctor had to increase my anti-nausea medicines, whose major side effect was the "C" word.

I have since tried several remedies to keep constipation in check: prune juice, milk of magnesia, stool softener, laxatives, Metamucil, and high-fiber foods. Dr. Moe has been vigilant in reminding me to take one or more of these correctives a few times each day. He has also kept a mental log (no pun intended) of my bowel movements. Though I appreciated his concern, I finally told him to stop asking me "Did you poop yet today?" in front of our children.

Since my current chemo drug, Taxol, is less nauseating than the drugs used during my first four infusions, I have needed fewer anti-nausea meds. I thought that would mean my troubles with the "C" word would be reduced, if not over. What fantasy world was I living in?

Up until yesterday, I was certain I preferred constipation to nausea and throwing up. I guess I still do, though I might not have said so on Sunday afternoon. Moe no longer needs to remind me to take my bowel remedies, any of which, incidentally, would make an excellent gift for someone starting chemo.

Postscript: After reading this post, sympathetic friends offered their own constipation remedies, including hemp seed and steel cut oats with ground flax seed. I also got some fun comments, such as, "Thanks for bringing a visual to 'sh–– a brick.'" and "I hope everything comes out okay—ha, ha!" For me, the most effective treatment was prescription lactulose, a synthetic, non-digestible sugar available in liquid form. I still keep some on hand, just in case.

Hike Therapy

Wednesday, November 9, 2011

One week after my fifth chemo, I am getting back to normal. The Taxol-induced body aches are gone, the fatigue is not so bad, and I am starting to get the "C" word (see last entry) under control. I was even able to go hiking with my girlfriends this morning for the first time in more than a week.

There were three of us on Piestewa Peak today, my two very fit pals slowing their steps to match the leisurely pace I must take up the mountain. Pace was not an issue this morning. We had stories to tell and problems to solve.

One of these friends, who lost her husband to cancer three years ago, is raising four teenagers on her own and doing an amazing job.

Every day she faces challenges in time management, transportation, disciplining, character building, and trying to provide her kids enough love for two parents. A while back, she threw dating into the mix, which has made her life even more complicated. We hear all about it on the mountain, where all of us vent, give and receive advice, and help each other feel better about our troubles.

The other friend on today's hike just returned from the funeral of her brother-in-law, a seemingly healthy fifty-seven-year-old whose heart gave out suddenly. This friend shared with us her sister's despair at losing the love of her life, the ripple effect of this man's loss in the lives of his children, stepchildren, and others who knew him, and the perceptibly endless details that must be attended to when someone dies.

I got my turn to talk, too, mostly about the adversities of my latest chemo. You readers are pretty familiar with those by now.

Resting at the top of the peak, the three of us agreed that losing a spouse and battling a life-threatening illness are two of life's worst events. What gets you through is the support of loved ones and friends, something my pal's sister is just finding out and I know very well. "That support is *everything*," I said, looking at two of my biggest supporters.

On the way down the mountain, it was the same old same old—tales of sick children, broken appliances, and family dramas. And you thought I went hiking just for the exercise.

Uncertainty Is a Constant

Friday, November 11, 2011

On Wednesday, I visited my oncologist for my first post-Taxol check-up and learned my white cell count was 42.3—a wildly high reading. My previous post-chemo white count (following Adriamycin and Cytoxan) was 2.2, and the normal range is 3.6 to 10.

I wasn't sure what to make of the high reading. *Low* white blood cell counts are often a serious side effect of Taxol. Some patients have to wait an extra week between infusions so their white cell count can recover. Apparently, that isn't going to be the case for me. "This means we can skip the Neulasta shot the day after chemo," my doctor said.

I liked the sound of that. I have mentioned Neulasta before, but just to review, it is a stinging shot in the arm that stimulates bone marrow to produce white blood cells. Neulasta's main side effect is bone pain, which combines in a not-so-nice way with the body aches that follow Taxol. (Incidentally, Neulasta costs an astounding $7,500 per shot.)

Another happy thought ran through my mind as I processed the news about my white cell count. "Does this mean I can eat salad tonight?" I asked. Uncooked vegetables and fruits are off-limits the week after chemo, when white counts typically are dropping.

"You can eat anything you want tonight," the doctor replied.

I've enjoyed a lot of salad the past few days, but another worry surfaced this afternoon. I got a message from the doctor's office saying that results from my liver enzyme test were high and to come in and repeat the test. Taxol is known to raise liver enzymes. If my tests aren't normal by next Wednesday, I may have to postpone the next chemo. I am hoping that won't happen but know I should be prepared. Uncertainty is a constant during cancer treatment.

Postscript: Following this post, my friend Gayle commented, "Uncertainty is a constant in life. We just live under the false assumption that we are in control." I believe she is right. Since cancer, I no longer live under that false assumption but sometimes wish I did. Uncertainty means I can't take anything for granted. Despite careful planning and my best efforts, I might not have tomorrow, or at least not the tomorrow I expected. This awareness makes me try harder to make each day, personal encounter, and choice count. Uncertainty makes me uncomfortable, but it also makes me live better.

A Walk to Remember

Sunday, November 13, 2011

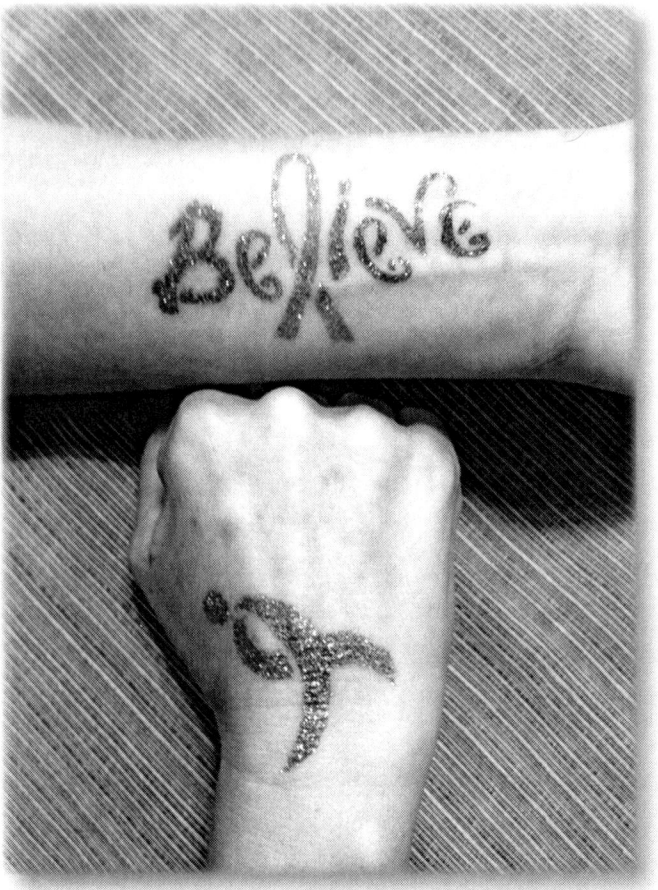

Above: My friend Robin, a fundraising dynamo for Crohn's disease, leukemia and lymphoma, and breast cancer, used her glitter tattoo kit to make me look like a breast cancer warrior.

Chemotherapy

This weekend, the Komen 3-Day Walk for the Cure took place very close to home, in north Scottsdale. I had mentioned to my friend Robin that I wanted to go see the walkers. Robin is a marathon runner recovering from knee surgery. We've been hanging out together lately, she in her wheelchair and me in a cotton cap to hide my baldness, playing Bananagrams and Scrabble at her kitchen table. A few days ago, Robin got cleared to start putting weight on her repaired knee, which meant she could ditch her wheelchair in favor of crutches and start driving a car again.

On the spur of the moment, Robin called yesterday and offered to drive us north to see the 3-Day walkers. She pulled up in front of my house like a convict who has just been released from hard time, an irrepressible smile on her face and the gleam of independence in her eyes. Ten minutes later, we were rolling along the event route, honking the horn at the sidewalk full of pink-clad walkers and support crews.

In a parking spot next to the route, Robin and I sat on her car's bumper clapping for each small group of participants that passed by. Some wore bright pink tutus, one male walker was dressed in drag, and others had pink-streaked hair, but most simply wore T-shirts covered with names of loved ones stricken with breast cancer. Some bounced along effortlessly, while others strained to keep going.

I choked down the lump in my throat and called out "Thank you" to each of them. I was moved most by the women whose shirts identified them as survivors, and by a male participant walking alone whose shirt said "Mom" in cursive beneath a large photo of a smiling middle-aged woman.

The 3-Day Walk is a big commitment. Each participant has to raise more than $2,000 and train to walk sixty miles over three days. Robin says they fudge the distance a little bit, and I've heard there is a bus that will pick up walkers who are too tired to continue. No matter. Each person who chooses to participate in the 3-Day Walk impresses me. Some day I hope to join their club.

Change of Plan

Tuesday, November 15, 2011

Sometimes things don't go according to plan. My sixth chemo treatment has been postponed until next week. My liver enzymes, while improving, are still elevated and the doctor wants them back in the normal range before nuking them with Taxol again. The nurse who gave me the news said, "You have a lot of years ahead of you and we want you to have a healthy liver."

I agreed, but couldn't hide my disappointment. I had hoped to be done with chemo by Christmas. That won't happen if I have to wait three weeks instead of two between each of the last three chemos. Oh well. Now I will have an extra week of feeling good. More days to hike and spend quality time with friends and family. More time to de-clutter the house and get a jump on my Christmas shopping.

While I would prefer to have chemo tomorrow instead of the day before Thanksgiving, I am already adjusting my attitude and expectations to accommodate the change of plan. I have to think about the big picture. We are on a cancer-killing mission here. As long as that job gets done, a few more weeks hardly matter.

Hard, but not Impossible

Thursday, November 17, 2011

This morning's hike up Camelback Mountain was the most difficult so far. It wasn't that my muscles hurt or my heart raced (though it did at times), but just that I felt tired. I shouldn't have been surprised.

Chemotherapy

My oncologist told me the effects of chemo would be cumulative and that I would feel increasingly fatigued.

I suppose I didn't want to believe him. Even when you know something is going to happen, it's not always easy to accept. While struggling up the trail, I lamented my slower pace and how much harder this climb is for me now. I doubted whether I should be on Camelback at all. It's the most strenuous of the regular hikes my girlfriends and I do.

When I shared some of these feelings with my friend Pam, she set me straight in a hurry. "I wonder how many people on chemo have hiked up Camelback," she said. "Not very many, I bet. You are doing great."

Our other pals were well ahead of us, hiking at their own pace, but Pam stayed by my side. She distracted me with stories and encouraged me on the steepest stretch of trail, where I was sorely tempted to sit down and call it a day. "Look," she said, pointing up the slope, "there is the saguaro cactus."

The tall, green desert sentinel, which appears to be growing right out of the rock, marks the spot where the trail turns left less than two-tenths of a mile from the top. If I could get to the saguaro, I knew I could make it the rest of the way. Pam knew it too.

Angie and Barclay were waiting for us at the summit and clapped when I arrived.

"Because you are still hiking, even slowly, you are going to bounce back like that after chemo," Barclay said, snapping her fingers.

Do I know how to pick my friends, or what?

When I got home, I thought about today's hike and how it was a metaphor for what I am going through right now. Enduring chemo, like hiking up Camelback, is hard but not impossible. You just have to believe you can do it and keep going at whatever pace your body will allow. A little help from your friends doesn't hurt.

Hot and Cold

Sunday, November 20, 2011

Over the past few weeks, as temperatures have cooled in Arizona and we have begun to use our thick comforter at night, my body has had trouble regulating its temperature. At bedtime, my feet, hands and nose are always cold. It takes several minutes under the covers before I warm up and fall asleep. My husband, whose metabolism is like a furnace, warms up immediately, and usually falls asleep within a minute.

For years Moe has teased me about my two-degree comfort range. According to him, if the temperature is 74–76 degrees, I am in heaven. Otherwise, it's either too hot or too cold. I used to argue the point but now just nod and say, "This is why we should consider a vacation home in Hawaii, the perfect climate zone for me."

Recently, something is different. I go to bed cold but wake up several times during the night hot, hot, hot. I'll be sweating and throwing off the covers one moment, only to be shivering and pulling the things back up five minutes later. Ladies, you know what I'm talking about.

It's happening during the day now, too. Sitting at my desk in the cool morning air with my jacket zipped up to my chin, all of a sudden a surge of heat will radiate through me. Next thing you know, I'm yanking the zipper down and throwing the fleece over the back of my chair. A few minutes later, I am chilled and scrambling to get the garment back on.

Considering my age, you might think hot flashes were already familiar to me. Well, they weren't. My oncologist said that chemotherapy would put me into menopause and that, at fifty-two, I would probably not come out of it afterward. Part of me doubted him, but the arrival of hot flashes and other symptoms have made menopause hard to deny.

Compared with the other byproducts of chemotherapy—nausea, baldness, fatigue, bone pain, low white blood cell counts, chemo brain, constipation, body aches, and elevated liver enzymes—hot flashes don't seem all that bad. You could say I'm hot and cold about the situation.

Sixth Chemo

Wednesday, November 23, 2011

Because my liver enzymes cooperated this week, I was able to have my sixth chemo infusion this morning, the day before Thanksgiving. When my oncologist saw me sitting in the chemo suite he came in to say hello.

"You didn't want to wait until after Thanksgiving, did you?" he said.

He understands my decision. I'd rather be a step closer to completing chemotherapy than feel good on the holiday. I'm very thankful not to have to wait *another* week.

I have to admit, the past week has been a pleasure. Following a chemo infusion, you feel better with each passing day, so the third week was even better than the second. With white counts in the normal range, I didn't have to worry so much about being exposed to illness. I hiked several times; went to a holiday light display at the Phoenix Zoo; accepted a dinner invitation with friends; and attended a meeting of my book group for the first time in months.

Despite some physical discomfort and minor annoyances (like having to give up wine until chemo is completely over), life is still pretty good three-quarters of the way through chemotherapy.

Six infusions down, only two to go.

Postscript: At times during chemotherapy, I desperately wished for a fast-forward button—like when the cancer drugs made me sick to my stomach, or the bone pain and body aches got to be too much, or the cool winter days made me miss my hair and the warmth it provides. In the last month or so of chemo, when the weeks dragged on and I just wanted it to be over, my mind fixed on finishing by a certain date—Christmas or thereabouts. Though the unpredictability of the chemo process meant I couldn't count on finishing "on time," having a deadline of sorts seemed to help. While not as good as a fast-forward button, it reminded me that chemo wouldn't go on forever. I only needed to hang in there for a little while longer.

Thanksgiving

Thursday, November 24, 2011

This holiday provides a reminder that gratitude is key to living well. While not thankful to be battling a life-threatening illness this year, I don't feel bitter or angry at the world. All of us have troubles in our lives—financial problems, family discord, health crises, loss of loved ones—and they never seem to come at convenient times. How we respond to these events, whether we learn from them and grow or become sour and defeated, defines the lives we lead.

It might sound weird, but I am grateful to cancer for making me grow. A cancer patient understands as never before that life is fragile and not to be wasted. Living in "the now" should never take a backseat to planning for the future, because now is for real and the future only a possibility. Such insights have made me quicker to acknowledge the important people in my life. They have prompted me to reexamine my spiritual beliefs and bring some definition to an area of my life that had been hazy for years. My disease has forced lifestyle changes, inflicted aches and pains, and demanded more flexibility than I would have thought possible. It has left me more determined than ever to lead a life that has meaning and a positive impact on the world. Thank you, cancer, for this new enlightenment. Let's hope it stays with me once I am cured.

Most of all this Thanksgiving, I want to acknowledge all of the friends and family members who are helping me through this trying time. Thank you to each person who has prepared a meal for my family. Thank you to the women in my bunko and book groups for their ongoing support. Thanks to everyone near and far who has sent a gift, card, or email message, or picked up the phone to call and cheer me on during this journey. Thank you to the army of medical people who are working so hard to help me and other cancer patients get better. I give the ultimate thanks to my front line of support, Moe, Brian, and Emily. No one fighting cancer ever had better backup, and I am deeply grateful.

When Lightning Strikes

Monday, November 28, 2011

A few weeks ago, I got an email from my high school friend, Jane, telling me that she had just become engaged. After a few decades in an unhappy marriage followed by a divorce, Jane had cautiously begun dating again a few years ago. "I want what you have," she told me, by which she meant a good man with whom to share the rest of her life.

Jane didn't find her ideal match right away. She spent a lot of time reflecting on what had gone wrong in her marriage before jumping into the choppy waters of online dating. Despite her new insights and determination to find love, she had a few false starts before finding a good match in Dan. Though he seemed to be everything she'd been looking for, she hesitated to make a commitment.

Jane and Dan had both failed at marriage before and didn't want it to happen again. To help them determine whether they were right for each other, they took a class for couples considering marriage. That experience only brought them closer.

When Jane and Dan got engaged, I was happy for my friend. She had traveled a long road on her way to Dan. Now, she would have what I have.

Last Friday, the couple's journey to happiness took an unexpected detour. Dan, an athletic nonsmoker in his fifties, suffered a major heart attack and had to undergo triple bypass surgery. Jane spent the weekend by his side, praying for his survival while at the same time thinking, "You've got to be kidding me, God."

By the time I spoke to Jane on Sunday, Dan had made it through surgery and already taken a short walk down the hall by his hospital room. Once she saw him alert and able to walk, my friend let go of her fears and once again pictured a future with Dan. She knows his damaged heart may slow him down, but feels certain they can still have the life they'd planned.

Sometimes life ignores the merits of your healthy lifestyle and threatens your existence with a heart attack, stroke, or cancer. It mocks a brilliant mind with the onset of dementia. It aims lightning bolts at unsuspecting hikers and sends cars driven by drunk drivers into the paths of innocents.

Whatever unfair crisis you are facing, the attitude you and your loved ones adopt will have a huge impact on your new reality. Will you go forward with determination and a positive outlook, or let despair and anger get the best of you? Will you focus on what you or a stricken loved one *can* do, or forever lament abilities that have been lost?

I already know which way Jane is going to go, and I'm glad. Her attitude is bound to have a healing effect on Dan's wounded heart.

I'm certain of this because an upbeat mindset has helped me overcome the travails of chemo. The day after my first infusion, when

I threw up for six hours straight, a phone call came from my former stepmother. Pat M. battled breast and colon cancer at the same time several years ago and has recently been dealing with a breast cancer recurrence. "The best thing you can do is be positive," said the cancer veteran. "It makes everything easier." As awful as I felt that day, Pat's message sunk in. I'm doing my best to heed her advice.

Postscript: Though they have yet to tie the knot, Jane and Dan have adapted to his ongoing health concerns and enjoy a rich life together. Pat M. is still going strong in her early eighties despite two localized recurrences of her breast cancer.

Dear Santa...

Wednesday, November 30, 2011

When my sixth chemo was postponed for a week due to high liver enzymes, the blues set in. I'd hoped to finish chemo before Christmas, but knew that would be impossible with three-week intervals between each of the last few treatments. Reluctantly, I adjusted my expectations.

Well, guess what? My liver enzymes didn't rise nearly as much following last week's sixth chemo infusion (my second encounter with the drug Taxol). This news came today during a doctor's appointment. The oncologist says I'll be fine to have my seventh infusion next Wednesday, December 7.

If my liver cooperates and I don't get sick and the sky doesn't fall, it's possible Chemo No. 8 (the last one) could still happen a few days before Christmas.

Santa, if you're listening, this is the gift I want most this year. (If that won't work, a few days after Christmas would be okay, too.)

Lessons from Ruth

Monday, December 5, 2011

On Friday, I had lunch with an eighty-nine-year-old woman I've known for decades but had lost touch with in recent years. A few weeks ago, having heard about my illness, she phoned to offer her support. Ruth had her own encounter with breast cancer twelve years ago. A lumpectomy, radiation, and five years on an estrogen-inhibiting drug brought her a cure. "I got through it and so will you," she said.

Ruth has endured health scares besides breast cancer and is currently nursing a painful worn-out knee. You don't get to be her age without learning to deal with adversity. Physically, she is not the same person I interviewed for a magazine article twenty-five years ago, when she was a successful realtor. These days she gets around with a walker or cane and her movements are slow. Mentally, she is as sharp as ever—possibly a little quicker on the uptake than her younger lunch companion.

Ruth doesn't drive a car anymore, but she still lives independently in the home she has occupied since 1969. Family and friends are a big part of her life, but not all of it. A talented fine artist, she still paints, knits, crochets, and teaches painting to students in her home. She also grows vegetables and flowers on her back patio, where she enjoys a view of Camelback Mountain that has not changed despite forty years of growth and transformation in the city of Phoenix.

I was happy to see Ruth living so well in her ninetieth year. "You are lucky," I said, thinking of my mother-in-law and the dementia that stole her away from us in her early eighties.

Ruth nodded in agreement. "I try to keep things light," she said. "Every Saturday night I watch the funny shows on PBS and I laugh."

What a great idea. Laugh, do the things you love to do, stay close with family and friends. I think this must be what *Star Trek's* Spock meant when he wished friends to, "Live long and prosper."

My Little Girl

Tuesday, December 6, 2011

Tonight Moe and I celebrate our daughter's eighteenth birthday. She is now legal to buy cigarettes, join the armed forces, and vote. She can go to adult prison, get a tattoo or piercing without our permission, and do other things I don't even want to mention. Fortunately, Emily has a good head on her shoulders. She usually displays good judgment and is responsible for very few of our gray hairs.

Emily arrived in the world weighing 11 lbs., 2 oz. She looked like a three-month old and was by far the largest baby in the hospital nursery. At first she had dark hair that all fell out, then no hair for almost a year before sprouting a crop of blonde curls to frame her smiling face and large green-blue eyes.

Our young child was sweet, affectionate, and put a lot of effort into everything she did. A sensitive soul, she was distraught to see any person or creature in distress. Emily soon charmed her parents. Bit by bit she even won over her older brother, who didn't like sharing attention with this interloper after three years as the only game in town.

Emily brought joy and balance to our family, and still does. She's a friend to everyone in the house, though not one to tell you what you want to hear at the expense of the truth. The hardest part about our "baby" turning eighteen is that she will not be in our house much longer. We are trying to enjoy every day between now and next fall, when she heads off to college.

This afternoon, I pulled my long, lean daughter onto my lap for some birthday TLC. She barely fit. Emily is a young woman now, five inches taller than her mom and mature beyond her years, but some part of her will always be my little girl.

Postscript: Emily remembers her eighteenth as the birthday when her mom was having chemo. We couldn't have a party because of my illness. Moe and I took her out to dinner but had to make an early night of it because I tired easily. There were presents but not much fanfare. I look back on that time and wish it could have been different. Though she must have been disappointed, our daughter didn't complain. She behaved like a grown-up.

Our girl's next birthday was much more carefree, shared with friends at college. Though we weren't there, it was hard to miss the party atmosphere in Facebook pictures she and her pals posted the next day. Those pictures made me smile.

Chemo Postponed

Wednesday, December 7, 2011

I arrived at the chemo suite this morning all set to have my seventh chemo infusion. It was not to be. Blood tests showed that my white cell count was critically low. The nurse gave me a shot of Neupogen, a short-acting medicine that stimulates bone marrow to produce white blood cells. We'll try again next Wednesday.

The chemo ride is full of highs, lows, dips, and curves. Sometimes it makes you sick, and just when you think you can't stand it anymore segues into a long, smooth straightaway. I didn't appreciate today's surprise, but I understand that passengers on the chemo express have little control. All we can do is roll with the ride and accept that it'll be over when it's over. In my case, not before Christmas, apparently!

Postscript: My memory of that day is still vivid. In the fourth month of treatment and nearing the end, another delay brought stinging disappointment. With my liver enzymes under control, I'd thought I was home free. Never did I expect my previously excellent white count to let me down. The frustration lingered for a few hours, until I thought of the many patients whose bodies can tolerate an infusion only every three weeks. For them, chemotherapy lasts for six months. By comparison, I was zipping through the process. During chemo, as in life, it's better to focus on what's going right than on the setbacks.

Warm Comfort

Saturday, December 10, 2011

It's December in Arizona and finally a little bit cold. Don't laugh. We desert dwellers spend seven months a year dealing with intense heat, so when nighttime temperatures dip into the thirties, it really does feel cold.

The temperature inside my house right now is a frigid sixty-eight degrees. "Frigid" might seem an exaggeration, but when you are bald, thin, and chemo-fatigued, you need a fleece jacket, hat, and blanket to be comfortable napping at sixty-eight degrees. Or maybe it's just me.

Fortunately, I'm seldom chilled. Thanks to some thoughtful friends, a blanket or wrap awaits next to each of my napping spots. A brown and blue rectangular prayer shawl with a decorative fringe, crocheted by Connie, drapes over the back of the living room couch. A plush tan throw embroidered at the corner with the word "Courage" and the pink breast cancer symbol lies folded at the foot of my bed. It came to me several weeks ago courtesy of five ladies who work in Moe's office.

Susan, whom I've known since our sons were in preschool, crocheted the green, blue, and off-white cotton blanket I keep near my recliner in the family room. "This is just something I made for you," she said shyly on presenting me the gift.

My newest wrap arrived this week from Washington, D.C. It is a vibrant blue triangular prayer shawl sent by Karen, a classmate who lived across the street from me during high school. Karen's friend Lisa, whom I have never met, helped Karen pick out the yarn and then knitted the shawl for me. Lisa's husband battled cancer six years ago so perhaps she felt some connection.

"We thought this design could serve as warmth and comfort as you undergo cancer treatments and, in years to come, as a fancy accessory for cool nights out on the town," Karen wrote in the accompanying card. "This shawl comes to you with all our prayers. A web of love and friendship knits us all together."

I use these coverings often. They are a soft armor of protection in my fourth month of chemo. They warm my body and also my heart. Every time I pull one over me, I think of the people who cared enough to provide them.

Postscript: I still pull on these wraps during cold weather. I've also kept the headscarves, hats, and a couple of pink hoodies that kept me warm during my bald phase. "Warrior" is emblazoned on the back of one jacket; "Hope! Fight! Cure!" is inked across the front of the other. At some point, I'll pass along the headgear and hoodies to other breast cancer patients, but can't imagine ever parting with the handmade shawls and blankets.

Psyching Up for the Next Phase

Monday, December 12, 2011

After chemo was canceled last week due to a low white cell count, I had Neupogen shots three days in a row. Today's blood test revealed that my white count is back in the normal range, so chemo looks like a go for this Wednesday. Barring further delays, my last chemo infusion will likely be the first week of January.

Though I still have two treatments to get through, my mind is jumping ahead to the next phase of this adventure. I meet with the breast surgeon at the end of December, a plastic surgeon who specializes in reconstruction in early January, and have a tentative surgery date of January 26. Nothing is set in stone, but plans are taking shape.

Over the past few months, surgery seemed so far away that I seldom thought of it. Now I think about it often and have a lot of questions. Has chemotherapy killed most of the cancer? Will I have radiation before or after reconstruction? Should I even have reconstruction (leaning toward "yes")? Will my left arm be damaged after lymph nodes are removed from the armpit? Will all of the surgery/recovery/radiation interfere with my hiking plans for next fall? (You can't take the hiker out of the cancer patient.) Oh yeah, and will I be cancer-free when all is said and done?

Some of those questions are unanswerable at this point. That last one is the biggie and troubles me most. I try not to worry about it. I'm getting excellent medical care and great support from friends and family. I'm following doctor's orders, doing all I can to stay healthy. I'm also trying to live in the "now."

Just the same, so much uncertainty and lack of control can be unnerving. In hopes that a strong will and desire have some impact on outcomes, I am dreaming of a future in which I get to know my (as yet unborn) grandchildren and grow old with Moe.

Finish Line in Sight

Thursday, December 15, 2011

Chemo No. 7 went off without a hitch yesterday afternoon. With only one more infusion to go, either the last week of December or the first week of January, I'm starting to envision the chemo finish line.

Later today, I'll have a shot of Neulasta, the long-acting bone-marrow stimulant, to boost my white blood cells for next time. Nurses at my doctor's office say the medicine will make it possible for me to have chemo in two weeks instead of three. I've heard that one before and won't get my hopes up.

Tomorrow, body aches from the chemo drug Taxol will set in and my activities will be limited for a few days. Between the chemo aches and the bone pain following a Neulasta injection, I may be a little grumpy this weekend. Maybe that's why Emily and Moe are heading north to our cabin, though it could be just to see the snow.

"Will you keep an eye on your mom while we're away?" Moe asked our twenty-one-year-old son when he emerged briefly from his man-cave bedroom this morning. Brian trained computer-weary eyes on his dad and nodded. He is a young man of few words these days, and sometimes all we get are grunts. He should be the perfect companion for me this weekend.

Joy of the Season Trumps Germ Phobia

Monday, December 19, 2011

Over the past few weeks, the peak of cold and flu season, I have thrown caution to the wind and attended some holiday gatherings. Since a fluctuating white count makes it impossible to know when I might be most susceptible to illness, the prudent thing would have been to stay home.

The prudent thing is not always the right thing. Sometimes you have to take some calculated risks and do what makes you happy. So, I went with Moe to his office holiday party, seeing some of his co-workers for the first time since losing my hair. Any self-consciousness I felt disappeared in well wishes and holiday cheer.

A few days later, I joined my bunko buddies for the December get-together no one wants to miss. We had a festive meal and then gathered for a few raucous games of Left, Center, Right. (We don't play bunko in December. Go figure.) Picture sixteen women at a large table, rolling special L, C, R dice and passing dollar bills up and down the line until all the money but a bill or two is piled at the center. The last woman with a dollar in front of her wins the pot. Try to imagine the squeals of delight and howls of disappointment that accompany this game, especially after the wine has been flowing.

December bunko was the most fun I'd had in weeks, and I didn't worry about germs once. When the room full of excited females became overly warm and I took off my hat to cool down, no one minded the sight of my naked head. There were even a few cheers. My bunko buddies have given me tremendous support these past few months, but this night I was just part of the gang, and it felt good.

The next week, my book group met for a holiday dinner and book discussion at Kathleen's house. An accomplished chef, she served the nine of us duck legs garnished with dried cherries over a bed of wild rice and grains. The dish tasted good even to my chemo-whacked taste buds. Others in the group brought appetizers, sides, and desserts.

These bookish women have provided meals for my family, offered to drive me to chemo, and called to cheer me up since my diagnosis in August. They knew just what to say and do, since I am not the first among us to cope with breast cancer. Liz, a native Scot and natural storyteller, went through the same ordeal in 2010. She now refers to that time as her "year of inconvenience." At the December dinner, Liz noticed that I had lost my eyebrows and lashes along with the hair on top of my head.

"I lost those, too," she said, raising her thick brows for emphasis.

For some reason, losing my brows and lashes bothered me more than losing my hair. While Christmas shopping, I have passed by mirrors and plate glass windows and wanted to cringe at the alien reflection. Seeing Liz with a full head of hair and completely restored brows and lashes made me feel better.

I've also taken note of her seize-the-day approach to life since she battled cancer. This fall she traveled to Vermont, Chicago, and Scotland to see people and places she enjoys. Between trips, she continues to work with the elderly and their families (as she did through cancer treatment). Liz, you are an inspiration to me.

I took some chances with my health in venturing out to these and other events during the holiday season. Perhaps I was emboldened by not contracting so much as a cold since starting chemo in early September. Or maybe my husband has given me an inflated view of the germ-killing powers of hand sanitizer. Either way, I'm glad I took these opportunities to be with good people celebrating the joy of the season. Without doubt, it was better for my health than staying home.

Postscript: Looking back, I was incredibly lucky. Somehow, despite my outings, a daughter in high school, and a husband treating cold and flu patients at work every day, I remained free of viruses and other infections during four months of chemo. Not everyone going through chemo will be so fortunate, but there is good medicine out there to treat whatever infections may arise. You just have to take things as they come, day by day, and know that eventually treatment will be over.

My Proudest Accomplishment of 2011

Monday, December 26, 2011

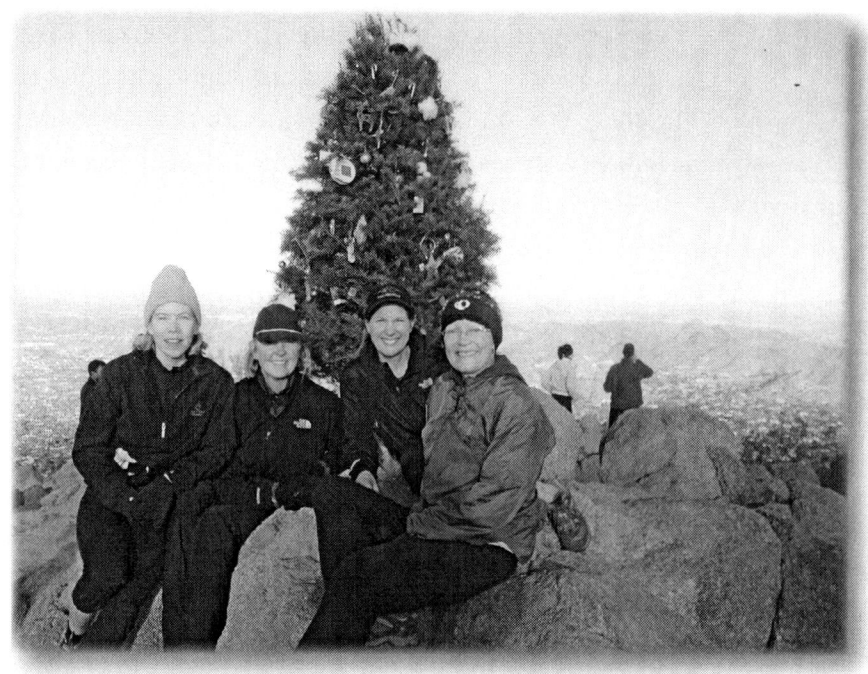

*Left to right: Barclay, Angie, Pam and me atop
Camelback Mountain on December 23.*

The past few years, it has become a tradition for the Obsessive Exercise Buddies—Barclay, Angie, Pam, and me—to hike up Camelback Mountain at Christmastime. Every year the mountain's regular hikers hang decorations on a tree atop the peak. Oftentimes it is a palo verde tree that grows out of the rock naturally. Other years, including 2011, it is an actual Christmas tree that zealous hikers have hauled 1,300 feet up the boulder-strewn slopes.

Throughout the fall, while progressing through chemo, I have worried that I might not be strong enough to make it up strenuous Camelback at the end of December. Following my seventh chemo treatment, on December 14, I was wracked with body aches for more than a week. I also had numbness in my fingertips and feet, a Taxol side effect I had not experienced previously. At night, the soles of my feet felt like they were on fire. The numbness/burning was due to chemo-induced nerve damage called "neuropathy," which can last for weeks, months, years, or forever.

How will I hike if I can't feel my feet? I wondered.

When I saw the oncologist last Tuesday, he had encouraging news. Since the neuropathy hadn't appeared until my second-to-last treatment, he felt certain it would not last. "It may take months to go away, though," he added.

The improvement in my feet between Tuesday and Friday is a testament to the human body's resilience. Each day, my knees became a bit steadier and my feet less numb. My friends knew Camelback might not be possible for me and offered to do our Christmas hike anywhere I wanted. On Thursday night, I told them I would give Camelback a shot. If it got too hard, I could always sit down and wait for them to finish the climb.

As you can tell from the photo on the previous page, I made it all the way up. It was a cold, breezy, and clear day that allowed us to see for many miles in every direction. Sharing the view and some hugs with my girlfriends was an awesome Christmas gift.

In the parking lot at the bottom of the mountain, my face broke into a big smile, as if I had just then realized how happy I was. "If you had told me in September that I was going to be on top of Camelback Mountain on December 23rd, I don't know if I would have believed it," I said to my friends.

Continuing to hike up mountains throughout chemo is perhaps my proudest accomplishment of 2011.

Postscript: The year I got cancer was one of the worst, and best, of my life. An excerpt from our holiday letter explains why:

> For our family 2011 has been a year with a split personality. In the beginning ... we spent months pouring over Rick Steves' guidebooks to plan a European adventure in July. The dreaming and anticipation were almost as delicious as the vacation itself. Almost.
>
> Emily and I spent the entire month of July traveling the Continent and had the time of our lives. For the first sixteen days, we were on our own, touring Rome, Siena, Florence, and the Cinque Terre in Italy, then Nice and Paris in France....
>
> For the second half of our adventure, we met Moe and Brian in Bruges, Belgium, and continued by car through Luxembourg, Germany, and the Czech Republic. In Germany, we followed the path Moe's late mother (a native German) traveled as she made her way home to Leipzig from Heidelberg at the end of World War II....
>
> Two weeks after we returned from our dream vacation, I was diagnosed with breast cancer. At first it seemed like the best-case scenario, a tiny tumor that hadn't spread. But an MRI indicated a larger mass that involved some lymph nodes. That's when our year went from Dr. Jekyll to Mr. Hyde....

Emily and I documented our European travels in a blog (europe onestepatatime.blogspot.com). At the end of each day, we posted our impressions and photos. When I was feeling low during cancer treatment, a visit to our Europe blog site was guaranteed to cheer me up. My second-proudest accomplishment of 2011 was planning and executing that trip, fending off pickpockets and overcoming language barriers along the way. Emily and I learned to think on our feet and adapt to conditions on the ground while still following our general plan—skills that came in handy during chemo and beyond.

Last Chemo Tomorrow

Tuesday, December 27, 2011

Tomorrow at 8 a.m. I will report to the chemo suite for the last time. I thought my white count would be too low or my liver enzymes too high to permit chemo this week, but the doctor's office just called to say I'm good to go.

Maybe I should be ecstatic, but I have mixed feelings. Still tired from the last chemo infusion and the excitement of Christmas, I feel unsettled about the future. The last chemo signals the end of phase one and the beginning of phase two of my breast cancer journey. Surgery is only four weeks away.

Until now, I've lost only my hair to this disease. In a month, I'll lose a part of myself that won't grow back (though it can be reconstructed). While I'm eager to get rid of the cancer, losing the breast is a different matter. I wish it didn't have to happen. Breast cancer has already changed my life, but soon the change will be more noticeable, at least to me. I plan to follow the example of many women before me who have gone through this ordeal, held their heads high, and gone on with their lives.

But first things first. I am finishing chemo tomorrow and will be sipping some champagne on New Year's to celebrate the achievement.

Chemo Is Done!

Wednesday, December 28, 2011

Early this morning, a nurse at the oncologist's office stuck a needle into the port in my chest to begin the premeds for my last infusion of Taxol. First a little bag of liquid Benadryl dripped into the vein near my heart, and then came an anti-nausea med. By the time the Taxol was dripping down the tube, the Benadryl had knocked me out. I awoke slowly two hours later with less than half the bag of Taxol to go.

The whole process took a little over four-and-a-half hours. At the end of an infusion, one of the nurses usually comes over to remove the needle from my port and send me home. It might be red-headed Angie with her Tennessee accent and warm smile; brunette Sherry, who's been a chemo nurse for twenty years and offers advice with a voice of experience; or olive-complexioned Lettie, whose big brown eyes beam empathy and understanding. Today, all three of them came to my chair and showered me with homemade confetti.

I smiled at them with tears in my eyes but could hardly speak. All the emotions of the past four months had welled up inside me. They had probably seen this reaction before. I wish I'd been better able to express my gratitude for the kindness and excellent care I received at their hands.

Although a week of body aches lies ahead of me, I feel like I've already made it through chemo. It wasn't always pretty (and I certainly don't feel pretty at the moment), but I'm still standing and perhaps a little more confident about overcoming the challenges ahead.

Postscript: A few months later, I peeked into the room where I'd had my treatments and realized something. The nurses who care for everyone never graduate from the chemo suite. They see a steady stream of patients afflicted by cancer: young, old, male, female, strong, and frail. Some who pass through the chemo suite are cured; others aren't, but gain precious time. A few respond poorly and have to stop chemo prematurely.

I think you'd have to have an enormous heart and rhino-thick skin to be a chemo nurse. Just taking on the job should be an ironclad guarantee that you'll never get cancer. Of course, it's not, but I have to believe there is a special place in heaven for those who choose to do this work.

SURGERY

3

"In the midst of winter, I found there was within me an invincible summer."

—Albert Camus

New Year's Wish

Sunday, January 1, 2012

I love New Year's Day. It is a legacy from my father, who raised me to be full of optimism and dreams on January 1. This morning, four days after my final chemo infusion, I set out on the hiking trail to ponder my aspirations for this year. The cobalt skies and sunlit spiny fuzz outlining each giant saguaro cactus along the path made me forget about my light muscle aches and the tingling in my hands and feet. It felt good to be in motion and making plans.

If 2011 was the year I got cancer, 2012 is the year I expect to become cancer-free. I have other goals, too—to hike the Grand Canyon again, for one—but getting rid of cancer is Job 1. To that end, Moe and I met with my breast surgeon last Friday to discuss the next stage of my treatment.

A friend of mine who had a lumpectomy in 2010 said she met with her surgeon for "maybe five minutes" prior to surgery. My surgeon spent a full hour discussing options with Moe and me when we first met with her last August. Talk about great first impressions. Dr. L.

is a positive spirit who loves her work and could teach her colleagues a thing or two about bedside manner. On Friday, she told me how great I looked after eight rounds of chemo.

"Some patients have trouble walking down the hall," she said, shaking her head. "You don't even look like you had chemo."

It sure felt like I had chemo, I thought to myself, while also appreciating the compliment. Like before, Dr. L. gave me a thorough examination and carefully explained my options. She could find nothing of the tumor we could all feel at the edge of my left breast last August. While that is very encouraging, she won't know until she operates just how much cancer remains in the breast and lymph nodes. I am opting for a "skin-sparing" mastectomy of the left breast, and will leave it to the doctor's judgment as to how many lymph nodes need to be removed.

If all goes well, after Dr. L. finishes the mastectomy, my plastic surgeon will enter the operating room to place a tissue expander under the remaining skin of the left breast, the first stage of breast reconstruction. After several weeks of healing, I will have radiation of my left armpit and chest area. Radiation should be finished by late April or early May. Roughly six months later, I will have the second phase of reconstruction.

There was a lot to think about while hiking up the Sunrise Trail this morning. It could have been overwhelming, but somehow wasn't. I know what is coming. I have excellent doctors and believe they'll do their best for me. I feel strong physically and emotionally. I've even come to terms with the fact that no one can assure I'll be cancer-free at the end of this long journey.

That's where Sunrise Peak comes in. I often hike there on Sunday mornings and have joked to friends that it's my "church of the mountaintop." Sitting on a rock looking out over greater Phoenix, I have sent up many a silent prayer, hope, and plea regarding problems that were beyond my control. This New Year's Day I sat on the mountain-top quietly articulating my concerns and wishes for 2012. Afterward, feelings of comfort and optimism washed over me, and I was not afraid of what lay ahead.

Strong Words

Thursday, January 5, 2012

Last January, my friend Gayle Nobel shared a powerful idea for the New Year. Gayle, whose twenty-eight-year-old son, Kyle, suffers from autism, writes inspirational books (*It's All About Attitude*, co-authored with Kathy Almeida, and *Breathe*), and a blog for families supporting a loved one with special needs.

In the eighteen years I've known them, Gayle and her husband, Neil, have endured many difficult times with Kyle while also raising two younger daughters. Their grace, stamina, and teamwork when under pressure have kept their family functional and their marriage strong. It hasn't been easy, but they have found ways to live well while also taking care of their son.

From Gayle I have learned that you can choose to be either a victim of, or victor over, your life's circumstances. As her book and blog titles say, "It's all about attitude." That is a powerful concept in its own right, but not the New Year's idea to which I was referring above.

Last January and again this year, Gayle encouraged her blog followers to pick ONE WORD as an intention for the New Year. A one-word intention is not the same as a resolution, she explained. It's not about solving a problem, such as losing weight, living within a budget, or being less critical of your spouse. Rather, it is a way to set a tone or create a mindset that will help you live better in the New Year. Here are some examples: laughter, compassion, nurture, move, stillness, patience, listen, forgive, breathe.

Last year, my word was "believe." I wrote it on a post-it note next to my desk, and it cheered me on through every hard task I attempted. The word "believe" erased my doubts that I could write fiction, plan and follow a complicated itinerary for a month-long foreign trip, and overcome the side effects of chemo.

"Believe" is now imprinted on a bracelet I wear. Since it's too good a word to give up, I've decided to amend Gayle's suggestion. Instead of one word, I will have two words for 2012. "Resilience" is my second word. It reminds me that when life knocks you down, you must get back up. "Resilience" is bound to help me through surgery, radiation, reconstruction, and whatever else this year throws my way. I urge you to select a touchstone word to remind you of your own intention for the New Year. I am grateful to Gayle for this idea and know she won't mind my sharing it with you.

Postscript: To get through hard times in life, it helps to have a well-stocked toolbox. I'm not talking about a receptacle of hammers and wrenches, but one full of mental, emotional, and spiritual implements that will help you stay focused and positive in the face of the biggest challenges.

During breast cancer treatment, my inner toolbox surprised me with its depth. Somehow the right device would float to the surface of my mind just when I needed it. I would think of an inspiring word, take comfort in a prayer on the mountaintop, find one thing to be grateful for on a most miserable day, remember to be present in each moment, or concentrate on putting one foot in front of the other even when the destination seemed unattainable. These tools got me through.

I continue to replenish my toolbox. You never know when you'll be confronted with something that requires you to dig deeply into it. An indomitable spirit is my sledgehammer.

Chemo's Forget-me-nots

Sunday, January 8, 2012

On Friday evening, I noticed a small cluster of itchy red bumps on my side between the ribs and hip. My family physician husband took one look and said, "You have shingles."

For the uninitiated, shingles is the adult version of chicken pox. If you had the childhood disease, you can get shingles later on. Though mostly a problem among the elderly, shingles can be triggered by stress or a weakened immune system and is not uncommon among chemotherapy patients. It can be just as itchy as the chicken pox and much more painful.

I had a mild case of shingles eleven years ago, perhaps due to stress from finding out I had pre-diabetes. "How many times can you get shingles?" I asked Moe incredulously.

"More than once," he said. "You should probably get the vaccine."

When I asked why he hadn't suggested this before, he explained that the shingles vaccine is still fairly new and has only recently been recommended for patients under age sixty.

Fortunately, the anti-viral medication Acyclovir can stop shingles in its tracks if taken within the first seventy-two hours of an outbreak. Moe knew this and contacted my oncologist, who called in a prescription. I have to take Acyclovir five times a day for a week, a small inconvenience for keeping the red bumps in check. My rash is still itchy but has not spread.

Meanwhile, I continue to experience tingling in my hands and feet as well as mild body aches. Those along with the shingles are little reminders that eight rounds of chemo toxins take a toll on your body while they are killing your cancer.

The Realities of Surgery in a "Plastic" World

Wednesday, January 11, 2012

On Monday, Moe and I met with my plastic surgeon in one of the more upscale doctor's offices I've ever visited: marble floors with mosaic inlays; front-desk countertop of cross-sectioned geodes accented by backlighting; deeply cushioned waiting room chairs upholstered in rich velveteen sporting the latest designer colors. I was glad I wore my "nice" jeans.

While waiting to be led back to a room, I couldn't help but notice promotional material hawking Botox, laser, liposuction, and a smorgasbord of other beautifying treatments. High-end cosmetic products were also on sale.

I was turned off by the fancy office and emphasis on female perfection. To me, beauty from the inside has always been more important than outer appearance, and this was especially true after months looking like a hairless alien. This place reminded me of all the feminine qualities that I am currently lacking.

Once inside a posh exam room, I noticed a table with a display of small, medium, and large breast implants. I poked a finger into the big one. "Wow," I said, smiling at my husband.

"That's got to be a D cup," he said, laughing.

Definitely not for me. I worried that the small one might even be too big to match my healthy breast. Moe assured me that implants come in other sizes besides the three on the table.

When Dr. G. entered the room, I made myself look past his designer suit and highlighted hair to focus on his words. What he said convinced me that, underneath the high-gloss façade, he is a highly skilled doctor.

The plastic surgeon patiently explained his role in my surgery. After the breast surgeon completes my mastectomy, the plastics specialist will enter the operating room to place a tissue expander underneath the remaining skin, reinforcing the area below the expander with sterilized cadaver skin. Over the ensuing four to six weeks, the expander will be injected with saline during office visits until it reaches the desired size.

For the first few weeks after the operation, chest tubes will be in place to drain fluids that build up after surgery. "During that time, you should avoid cardiovascular exercise," the doctor said.

"I'm a very active person," I interrupted. "How long after surgery until I can hike?"

"After six weeks, you can do anything you want," he said.

"What about during those six weeks?"

The look on his face indicated that this was not a typical question. "If you get your heart rate up while the tubes are in, you'll keep building up fluid and I won't be able to get the drains out. So, no cardio exercise for at least two weeks. After the drains are out, you can start walking."

The doctor measured my chest to determine the size for my tissue expander while I tried to get my head around the unpleasant realities of surgery. Pain, I could tolerate, but inactivity, not so much. I could go two weeks without exercising, I decided, but I would not be sedentary for six weeks. Not unless I was in a coma.

"Patients call this thing 'the rock,'" the doctor said, holding up the skin-colored plastic expander. Flat on the bottom and rounded on the top, the disk-shaped device sported small flaps on either side to help it stay in place, and a small port at its center to receive the saline injections. Dr. G. said that "the rock" would be in my chest through radiation treatments and for another eight to twelve months afterward, until my radiated skin is sufficiently recovered to permit successful reconstruction.

Using my mental calculator, I realized it would be December 2012 at the earliest before Dr. G. agreed to swap out "the rock" for a more comfortable implant. My breast cancer treatment/reconstruction adventure will not be ending anytime soon.

The next step is surgery, now scheduled for February 2.

Postscript: During that first visit to the plastic surgeon's office, I wished there had been a separate entrance and waiting area for cancer patients—a comfortable room without advertisements on elective procedures, where someone still recovering from chemo wouldn't feel so self-conscious.

While my biggest concern was survival—and, very secondarily, to have a normal bust line if I did survive—this medical practice seemed to be all about image. It was a poor fit for someone like me, but I stayed for one reason: By all accounts, the doctor was a breast reconstruction whiz who got excellent results.

My concern about inactivity following surgery seems silly in retrospect. After months of treatment, my patience was wearing thin. Staying active through it all had helped me cope physically and psychologically. I wasn't looking forward to "down time," and didn't feel well understood by the doctor, whose usual customer seemed so different from me. In the end, I listened to his advice, but also trusted my own instincts regarding the pace of my recovery.

A Little Bit of Normal

Tuesday, January 17, 2012

Between chemo and surgery, I have been craving a little bit of "normal." A few weeks in which I could regain my strength, cook my own food, and take a few weekend trips.

Last weekend, when I was less than two weeks post-chemo and still aching a lot, Moe took me on a mini-getaway to the scenic far-west side of metropolitan Phoenix. More specifically, we drove to a farmer's field in the middle of nowhere to look for a bird, the Smith's longspur. Following directions from a birding web site, we pulled up on the edge of a dirt road next to the field, and saw a dozen people in the distance bent over spotting scopes attached to tripods.

"They're on the bird," Moe said excitedly. He hopped out of the car, grabbed his own scope from the trunk, and strode quickly across the field to join the group. I followed closely on his heels. Two minutes later, we were enjoying our own magnified view of a small brown bird perfectly camouflaged in the dry grasses of the fallow field.

Back in the city, my husband took me to lunch and then for a long walk by a scenic manmade lake where he could, incidentally, scan the surface for water birds that winter there. We spent the whole day outside, enjoying the simple pleasures of a sunny winter's day.

This past weekend, we ventured farther from home, to the western edge of Arizona. Once again, we were chasing rare birds. Moe spotted eight Barrow's goldeneye at Bill Williams Nature Preserve, a Thayer's gull at Lake Havasu, and the most spectacular winged creatures of our trip, five trumpeter swans, in a field north of Needles, California.

The swans, five feet long from beak to tail, had flown south all the way from the Arctic. Like 747s, these big flyers burn a lot of fuel in the air, and fed nonstop from muddy puddles in the field as we observed them.

We spent Saturday night in Lake Havasu City, a sprawling community defined by RV, car, and boat dealerships; lakeside marinas and resorts; and strip malls by the dozen. The most elegant structure in town is London Bridge, disassembled in England and reassembled here in the late 1960s.

In warm weather, Lake Havasu is clogged with boats, but in chilly January, the waterway is a quiet sanctuary for birds. It's also a great time to get a discounted accommodation with a view. From our room's balcony on Sunday morning, we saw the sun rise over the glassy lake, jagged mountains jutting up on the right, civilization spreading along the shore on the left, and a healthy avian population diving for breakfast in the water below.

How nice it was to wake up in this different world, far away from thoughts of cancer, chemo, and surgery, and feel a little bit of normal.

The Luck of Moe

Thursday, January 19, 2012

At least once a week, my health-conscious husband rides his bike eight miles from our house to his office near Old Town Scottsdale. He travels through the park on a bike path most of the way, so I don't worry about it too much.

One time, about ten years ago, he ran into a curb he couldn't see in the dim morning light, flew off his bike and rolled onto the pavement like a tumbler, landing on his feet. The front wheel of his bike was destroyed, but he suffered only a small scrape and wounded pride.

Yesterday, about an hour after Moe pedaled off from our house, he called me from work. "You're going to have to pick me up at the end of the day," he said in a strange, amped-up voice.

"Why?"

"I had a wreck on my bike," he admitted sheepishly.

My first thought was that it couldn't have been too bad if he was able to call me. But actually, it *was* pretty bad. Moe had been following closely behind another (younger) rider on the bike path when they entered the underpass beneath Camelback Road going 20–25 mph. In the shadowy underpass, Moe saw the other guy swerve to avoid something. He couldn't see the two steel shopping carts that were blocking the path until just before he plowed into one of them.

Moe felt a sharp, electric pain on the left side of his ribs, and then he was in the air. Seconds later, he slid across the pavement on his left side and back. His helmeted head bounced back against the cement as he came to a stop.

The other biker heard the crash and returned to help. He and Moe disentangled Moe's bike from the shopping cart. Pumped up with adrenaline, Moe put the chain back on his heavily damaged bike and pedaled it the short distance to his office.

"I think I broke a rib," he told me. "And my knee, ankle, and wrist on the left side are starting to hurt."

I knew he wouldn't last the day and was unsurprised when he called before noon to ask for a ride home. In the car, Moe talked about how fortunate he'd been to walk away from the accident. Yet another example of "The Luck of Moe," we agreed.

A friend coined the phrase when Moe narrowly escaped catastrophe a few times during college. Like when the wheel of his car sheared off in the dorm parking lot at the end of a 400-mile drive from Arizona to Los Angeles. Or the time he caught his foot in the barbed wire at the top of a fence while hang gliding, and ended up dangling upside down from the wire instead of crashing into the ground.

This morning my resilient husband was sore but feeling well enough to go to work. He is a lucky fellow, but a tough one, too. Assuming The Luck of Moe extends to his wife, I have yet another reason to believe that I am going to be okay. I held onto that thought later in the morning, when we met with my radiation oncologist, and talk of surgery, another MRI, and six-and-a-half weeks of radiation burst the bubble of normalcy I've been living in lately.

I'd Rather Be on the Beach…

Monday, January 23, 2012

My breast cancer treatment involves four doctors—medical oncologist, breast surgeon, plastic surgeon, and radiation oncologist—and I have seen them all over the past few weeks. Our visit with the radiation oncologist last Thursday brought home the fact that my treatment is far from over. I left her office with complete confidence in my doctor, but sobered by what lies ahead. The post-chemo high was fun while it lasted.

Today, I had an EKG and lab tests to make sure my heart and major organs are healthy enough for surgery. Tomorrow morning, I will have an MRI that will give us some idea of how well chemo worked against my cancer. It will also provide the radiation oncologist with information she needs to create my treatment plan.

Tuesday afternoon, I will return to the plastic surgeon's office for more pre-op instructions. On Wednesday, I will be fitted for a camisole and special bras to wear after surgery. I've also been advised to acquire some loose-fitting blouses to wear over the bandages and drains that will surround my chest following the operation.

The schedule (which could change) is as follows: February 2, mastectomy (left side only) and placement of a tissue expander. Between February 2 and March 1, saline will be injected into the expander until it reaches the desired size. Around March 1, radiation begins, five days a week for six-and-a-half weeks. Radiation will target the left armpit, chest area above the breast, and mastectomy scar.

Providing all goes well, I will be done with treatment before my daughter's high school graduation in late May. In June, Moe and I will travel to Hawaii for a "Thank God it's over!" vacation. I have a feeling I'll be spending much of February, March, and April dreaming of the beaches of Kauai.

A Day to Remember

Tuesday, January 24, 2012

When you undergo cancer treatment, there are certain dates you will always remember. On August 15, I got my diagnosis. On September 2, I had my first chemo infusion, and on December 28, my last. I didn't expect to have another memorable day until surgery on February 2, but life surprises you sometimes.

Today, I had my second MRI and sailed through it. During my first MRI in August, forty-five minutes with my arms extended over my head in that deafening machine seemed like eight hours. My left shoulder cramped up halfway through and I had to use all of my mental tricks to make it to the end. Today, I knew what to expect and made sure I was comfortable, with my arms at my sides, before they rolled me into the magnetic noisemaker. Forty-five minutes felt like twenty minutes. I left Outpatient Radiology patting myself on the back.

Several hours later, Moe called from his office to ask permission to access my MRI report on the hospital computer. With some trepidation, I told him to go ahead. My first MRI had been a nightmare. It showed that the cancer in my breast was far more extensive than we'd thought, with disease in the lymph nodes as well. I hoped with all my heart that today's findings would be different and that somehow chemo had wiped out all of my cancer, but I knew it might not be the case. Moe had told me complete resolution only occurs in roughly one-fourth of patients.

Well, guess what? This afternoon, Moe read and re-read my MRI report before sharing the good news with me—my cancer is no longer detectable on MRI. The masses that were present in August are gone! This is the best possible outcome following chemo and improves my long-term prognosis. It's still possible that some cancer cells will appear under the microscope when tissue from my breast and a few lymph nodes are examined following surgery, but radiation should eradicate them. I am not yet cured, but things are looking up.

When Moe relayed this news, we both shed tears of relief. I couldn't wait to tell Emily and Brian. Chemo's success is a giant leap in my battle against breast cancer. I can hardly believe it and am trying to temper my excitement until I get official word from the doctors on my case. Thank you to everyone who is praying for me—I think it's working. January 24, 2012 is a day of hope I will always remember.

Postscript: My friend Barclay commented, "Shedding a few tears here, too. Congratulations! That's wonderful news."

My pal Gayle wrote, "Awesome, awesome, awesome news!!! Can't wait to celebrate with you."

No cancer detectable on MRI following chemo was awesome news, and it made me believe I might be cancer free. What an emotional high that was. *You got a really bad cancer, but it looks like you beat it!* I told myself. The future suddenly looked a whole lot brighter. My husband thought so too, even though he's in medicine and knows how imperfect MRI readings can be. Sometimes we believe what we want to believe.

A Dentist's Office That Makes You Smile

Saturday, January 28, 2012

On Thursday I went for a dental cleaning. Though people tend to put off this task, it had been seven months since my last dental visit, and I couldn't wait for Vicky the hygienist to make my fuzzy teeth feel smooth again.

Dental cleanings are not allowed during chemotherapy. The doctors don't want bacteria from your mouth traveling through your bleeding gums into your bloodstream when your immune system is weak. At the same time, the "dry mouth" that often occurs with chemo can wreak havoc on your teeth and gums.

I was worried about the condition of my mouth but forgot my concerns when Vicky spotted me in the waiting room. Her face creased into a broad smile and she welcomed me as if I were a hero just back from a war.

I don't know her secret, but somehow it never hurts when Vicky cleans your teeth. While she prodded and scraped inside my mouth with sharp metal instruments, she told me she had read my cancer blog and the other one Emily and I wrote about our trip to Europe. She paused often enough in her work so that we could have a conversation—about cancer, travel, family, and particularly our daughters, who are both high school seniors.

Before I knew it, my teeth felt silky again and Vicky had graded the condition of my gums "excellent." A little while later, my dentist, Dr. T., did his exam and gave the same rating. They both congratulated me on doing a great job of dental hygiene during chemo. Dr. T. told me he'd seen another chemo patient recently who hadn't been so fortunate. She had a decayed tooth that needed pulling, but her oncologist said her weakened immune system made the procedure too dangerous.

I don't know which made me feel luckier—that I wasn't that other chemo patient, or the big hug I received from Dr. T. before I left his office. "We all love you and we're glad you're doing so well," he said.

I went out the door with a bright smile.

Anticipation

Wednesday, February 1, 2012

The day before my mastectomy I feel much like I did prior to giving birth to my first child. I don't know exactly what it will be like, but

I do know that many women have gone through it before me and come out just fine.

In anticipation of a sedentary lifestyle during the few weeks after surgery, I've exercised madly for the past several days, huffing up the slopes of my favorite peaks, power-walking the bike path in the park, and power-cleaning my house. My errands are done, my overnight bag is packed, and I'm tired.

Maybe that means I will get some sleep tonight. My exhaustion is not just physical. As major surgery approaches, one tends to reconsider each decision. Are you sure you want a mastectomy and not a lumpectomy? Are you sure you don't want the healthy breast removed, too, so you never have to go through this again? Are you sure breast reconstruction is right for you? My answer to all of these questions is the same: Yes, I am sure (most of the time). No more second-guessing.

In recent days I've also been grappling with the emotions that rise up when one faces losing a body part. In the full-length mirror in our bathroom, nothing looks amiss with my chest. Cancer has not left any visible marks on my left breast. It is almost inconceivable that I will come home from the hospital on Friday without it. This reality makes me sad, but I'm making peace with it. A breast is a small price to pay for survival (and perhaps even a long life). Having a husband who will love me with or without mammary glands makes the loss easier to accept.

A big thank you to each person who has called, e-mailed, prayed for me, and sent cards and gifts this week. When I enter Piper Surgery Center for my mastectomy tomorrow morning, I will be riding high on a wave of your good wishes. And like so many brave women before me, I will get through it.

The Morning After

Friday, February 3, 2012

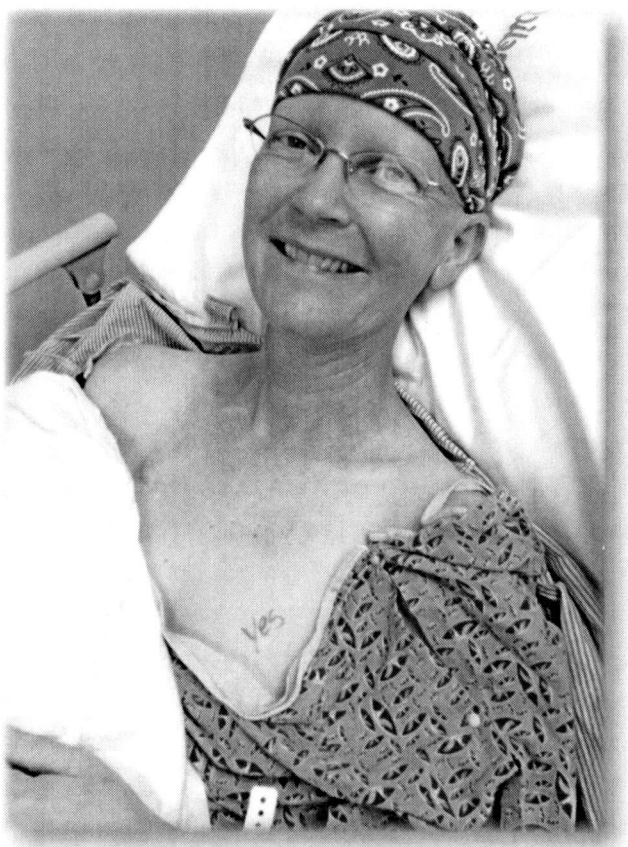

The past twenty-four hours have been a whirlwind. Moe and I arrived at the surgery center at 5:30 a.m. yesterday for a surgery scheduled at 8:45. I had to get signed in and gowned up before going to the far side of the hospital for an injection of radioactive dye. A nurse wrote the word "yes" at the upper edge of my left breast. I joked with her that she should add "no" on the right side.

Back at the surgery center, we had to wait more than an hour for the dye to move down to the sentinel lymph nodes that would be biopsied during surgery. Our children, Brian and Emily, had arrived by then, and we were all gathered in a pre-op room for a while. Nurses inserted an IV into my arm and all my doctors—anesthesiologist, plastic surgeon, and breast surgeon—came by to explain what they would be doing. The plastic surgeon marked my breast where he intended to cut and showed me where my scar would be.

Right before surgery, I received the margarita-like sedative the anesthesiologist had promised, and I was out cold for the next several hours. When I awoke in a private room upstairs, Moe told me the good news. The sentinel node biopsy showed no cancer. The breast surgeon removed only four lymph nodes. This was the best-case scenario. Moe was smiling, his face full of relief as he talked.

I might have smiled, too, but I don't remember. The lights went out again for me very quickly. I couldn't stay awake for more than a few minutes at a time for the next ten hours. Moe was worried, but it was only an effect of Phenergan, a strong anti-nausea drug and sedative.

This morning I feel great in spite of the pain in my chest. Surgery is over and no sign of cancer. Talk about a mood enhancer.

Postscript: In some respects, surgery is harder on family members than the patient. While I was anesthetized, my husband and children waited and worried. Whatever happened, they were powerless to help me. When I finally awoke from the ten-hour pain killer/sedative, my husband was far more stressed out than I was. He'd stayed awake all night, "to make sure you didn't stop breathing from the sedative." Moe got me home, where he could have some control over my recovery, as quickly as possible.

Gifts from Friends and Strangers

Sunday, February 5, 2012

On Friday, a man arrived at our door hefting the largest and prettiest floral bouquet I have ever received. It was from Rob and Julie, our longtime friends from California. When they called to order the flowers from a shop in Arizona, they told the woman on the line about my mastectomy. She'd had a sister with breast cancer and said she would make a special arrangement for me. When I look at it, I see inspiration and love. Thank you, R & J.

When Moe brought in our mail on Friday evening, there was a large envelope addressed to me. Inside I found a card and a long-sleeve T-shirt from a woman I knew during college but haven't seen in thirty years. After learning about my cancer in our holiday letter, a mutual friend put me in touch with Lindsay, who waged her own war against breast cancer about five years ago. Over the phone and in e-mails, Lindsay told me her cancer story, answered my questions, gave some sage advice, and helped me feel less anxious about surgery and reconstruction.

Lindsay's card brimmed with encouragement. On the front, beneath a drawing of a bird, it said, "The warbler sings his first notes upside down." Inside, she wrote, "You will find yourself upside down for a bit, but your path to healing will be easier because of your commitment to being up and out. Camelback awaits your return." A silk-screen design on the front of the shirt she sent features snow-capped peaks above the phrase, "I Like Mountains." Thank you, Lindsay, for helping me believe I will get my life back.

These are only a few examples of the touching gifts I've received recently. It seems like everyone I know has made an effort to support me in some way. I am indebted to them, and also to the people

I don't know very well (or at all) who have reached out to me simply because of our breast cancer connection. All of these helping hands have lifted me up during one of the hardest times in my life. I hope to do the same for others in the future.

Postscript: Lindsay was right—I did find myself "upside down" for a bit following surgery. In addition to physical discomforts, my emotions seesawed up and down depending on the latest test results. During those weeks, I imagined being in the mountains, by the beach—anywhere but in a medical office. Most of all, I envisioned (and hoped for) a future time when this would all be behind me.

Not for the Faint of Heart

Wednesday, February 8, 2012

I came out of surgery last Thursday with my chest wrapped in an Ace bandage. The next day, the plastic surgeon let me peek underneath it. I expected to see a flat space bisected by a scar on the left side of my chest. Instead, there was a small mound where the tissue expander he inserted following my mastectomy was already partially filled.

I also noticed three tubes connected to my chest. One skinny tube was attached to a pump that bathed my wound in a liquid painkiller. The other two led to drains that captured the seepage that occurs following a mastectomy. The drains are clear, hollow bulbs the size of a small fist. I have to drain them four times a day and record how much fluid they've collected.

For the first five days after surgery, I wore a small nylon bag around my neck to hold the painkiller pump, and a camisole with pockets on the side to hold the drains. I took a few pain pills (Vicodin) to keep me comfortable, and antibiotics to prevent infection. Though far from normal, the first days after surgery went far better than I expected. I could only sleep in one position, on my back with my head and shoulders elevated, but at least I could sleep. I couldn't hike, but felt good enough to walk around the neighborhood every day after returning home.

Yesterday, a nurse at the plastic surgeon's office removed two of the tubes. It took quite a bit of tugging to get the skinny painkiller tube out of my chest, and I nearly fainted at the end. There is something creepy about seeing twelve to eighteen inches of tubing emerge from your body, and it doesn't feel good, either. The experience left me lightheaded and queasy. The nurse had me lie down for a few minutes before pulling out one of the drain tubes. That one came out more easily and I was careful not to look at it.

As I stood by the front desk making my next appointment, the nausea returned and my vision went dim. Fortunately, I was not alone. My mother helped me to a chair, where I took deep breaths and waited for the feeling to pass. Mom and her significant other, Ed, are visiting Scottsdale this week to help us out. Since I'm not allowed to drive yet, they are taking me to appointments.

Later this morning, I'll visit my breast surgeon, who should have the pathology report on the tissue removed during my mastectomy. On MRI and in the lymph node biopsies, no cancer was found. I'm hoping the trend continues, but I know better than to count on it.

Reality Check

Thursday, February 9, 2012

In a perfect world, when no cancer has been detected in your pre-surgical MRI or in the frozen section biopsies of your lymph nodes, the pathology report based on a careful examination of all tissue removed during surgery would say, "No cancer anywhere."

Yesterday, I was once again reminded that we don't live in a perfect world. "It's a good thing you decided on mastectomy instead of lumpectomy," said my breast surgeon as she entered the exam room. She held my not-so-perfect pathology report, which said that chemo had killed most of the cancer, but not all of it.

In the breast tissue, the lump I found last winter at the 1 o'clock position had shrunk to 1–2 millimeters. Considering that its size was estimated at 2–5 centimeters prior to chemo, that's a very good result. A lumpectomy would have taken care of that spot. It would have completely missed a second 1.2-centimeter tumor located at 3 o'clock. It's surprising that my recent MRI didn't detect this second mass, but in the real world even our best technology has limitations. Microdots of cancer were also found in three of the four lymph nodes removed.

At first I was upset by this news. The past six months have been a roller coaster ride like no other. Good and bad test results, lengthy treatments, side effects, raised expectations, dashed hopes, uncertainty, worry, and fear all have been features of my heart-pounding breast cancer ride. Each time I have read a report stating the facts of my case, it has brought me down. This time, terms such as "invasive ductal carcinoma," "Nottingham grade 3," "positive superficial margin" and "micrometastatic disease" struck terror into my heart.

After taking a deep breath and reflecting on the big picture, I felt a bit better. Here is the good news: All the residual cancer found in my breast tissue and lymph nodes is *gone*. Any unseen, tiny cancer cells that may remain in the breast area or armpit will be nuked by radiation in a few short weeks. Thank God for effective breast cancer treatment. I am glad I listened to the inner voice that told me to have a mastectomy. In the real world, where there is much uncertainty and no guarantees in battling this scary disease, I appear to be winning the fight. It's not a perfect situation, but I'll take it.

Postscript: Have you ever awoken from a falling dream having just sailed over the edge of a cliff? That's the feeling I had on hearing the breast surgeon's recap of my pathology report. Beating cancer requires killing *all* the cancer cells. If you don't get them all, the cancer will come back, maybe not right away, but eventually. We were relying on three weapons to eradicate my aggressive cancer: chemo, surgery, and radiation. The pathology report told me that chemo and surgery might not have been enough (or possibly it was the look on my husband's face after he saw the report). Some stray cells might still remain in the breast skin, the lymph nodes, or even elsewhere in my body. I would have to count on radiation to finish the job, followed by years of estrogen-blocking medication. I might also need some luck and the grace of God.

Suddenly the clean MRI from two weeks before seemed like a cruel joke. The message inside my head went from *You beat cancer!* to *Only time will tell*. The anxiety I had begun to shed came back in full. As a friend put it, "A question mark hangs over your head." It wasn't the worst thing that could have happened, but it was a big letdown after being led to believe I might be home free.

While disappointed, I reminded myself that a question mark hangs over everyone's head. Circumstances had just made me more aware of it—and perhaps more motivated to live my best life in the present moment.

Six Months of Hard Time

Wednesday, February 15, 2012

Six months ago today, I was diagnosed with breast cancer. In the cosmic scheme of things, six months is no time at all. In the micro scheme of one person's life, it can seem like a very long time, especially when that person is fighting cancer.

When I mentioned the six-month milestone to my daughter, she suggested we celebrate. Though I understood her thinking—our family has dealt with the pressures of my illness admirably—a celebration didn't feel right to me. Not yet. We have made it through a hard six months. I am proud of my family and even a little bit proud of myself. With much support from friends and extended family, we have hung in there. Life has gone on around here without too much whining.

Valentine's Day, the eve of my half-year mark with cancer, brought mixed emotions. On the one hand, I've never felt more loved. On the other, I've seldom felt so uncertain. Though I have tried to be strong and positive, I couldn't stop the tears from welling up. Some of them were inspired by gratitude for the dozen roses and loving card I received from my husband. Others were the result of anxiety and weariness I experienced at the doctor's office, where we spent part of yesterday afternoon discussing my upcoming radiation treatments.

I wasn't worried about radiation. It shouldn't be bad compared with what I've already endured. I was more troubled by the discrepancy between the clean MRI before surgery and the not-so-clean pathology report that followed. One week I was led to believe all my cancer had melted away during chemo; the next week I found out micro traces of cancer had been found in a few lymph nodes as well as one significant mass in the breast that was removed. "What does it mean?" I asked the radiation oncologist.

She knew what I was getting at: How would this affect my long-term prognosis? "We don't really know," she answered, "but I think your chances are great for a good outcome. And I'm not just saying that." She gave several reasons: My cancer was very responsive to chemo, all the cancer seen under the microscope had already been removed, and radiation is very effective in killing any tiny clusters of cancer cells that might remain.

I had heard all of this before, but then the doctor added another factor in my favor—my lifestyle. Nonsmoking cancer patients who eat healthy foods, maintain a normal weight, and exercise regularly have lower recurrence rates.

I went into the doctor's office still sore from my recent surgery, and discouraged by the pathology report. I left the office with enough reassurance to refuel my positive attitude.

Postscript: My friend Gayle commented, "I think a positive attitude is another factor in your favor. Your emotional lifestyle is as important as your physical one. So breathe, smile, laugh, dust yourself off when you have the low moments, and continue on."

Those are words to live by, and I am trying to do so, even when the specter of cancer makes me doubtful about the future. Early this year my husband and I planned a special vacation months in advance. I insisted that we purchase trip insurance, something we never would have considered prior to my illness. While it might seem pessimistic to hedge bets in case my cancer comes back, the insurance brought me peace of mind. I think that's okay. What's not acceptable is to let fear diminish your life. My emotional lifestyle is built on positive expectation, humor, and curiosity about the world, which prevent me from sitting around waiting for the other shoe to drop.

Mixed Messages

Sunday, February 19, 2012

The doctor placed one hand against the side of my chest, where the tube emerged, and grasped the tube with the other. "One, two, three," he said, and pulled it out.

"That hurt," I said, gasping. Several other choice words ran through my head, and for a brief moment I felt like kicking him in the shins, or in a more sensitive place. Fortunately, the impulse passed quickly.

I had waited twenty minutes in the exam room before the plastic surgeon arrived to inflict this pain on me. While I caught my breath and reminded myself how nice it would be not to have to empty the drain that had been attached to the tube, the doctor admired the healing incision along the top of my partially expanded fake breast.

"Looks great," he said, noting that it would be ready for more expansion in a week or two.

Silent alarms went off in my brain. This was Friday afternoon. Three days prior, the radiation oncologist had told me we would start my radiation treatments by March 1. A CT scan, required for the planning of radiation therapy, was scheduled for next Friday. I needed to be fully expanded before having the CT scan.

My plastic surgeon frowned as I explained the time frame. "I've never heard of someone starting radiation less than six weeks after surgery," he said. "You need more time to heal."

My chest still throbbed, and I hadn't expected I would need to defend the treatment plan to one of my physicians. The breast surgeon and radiation oncologist both had said radiation should start by the fourth week post-surgery. Why was this news to my plastic surgeon? Would something go terribly wrong if I started radiation so soon?

"We don't want my cancer to come back," I told the plastics man. He acknowledged his work had to take a backseat to my cancer treatment, and we set my next appointment for two days before the CT scan. But the doctor had planted seeds of worry that sprouted as I left his office. What if my incisions opened up during radiation and refused to heal? What if we delayed radiation and unseen specks of cancer grew into life-threatening tumors?

It took some effort to rein in my imagination. When I had it under control, I realized it's up to me to listen to my doctors and ask questions until I am satisfied that my treatment plan minimizes risks. Ideally, all of my doctors would meet regularly to discuss my case. Each would know what the others were thinking and doing. In reality, that doesn't happen.

So, this week I will be contacting my doctors once again to make sure we are all on the same page.

From Needless Worries to Happy Trails

Friday, February 24, 2012

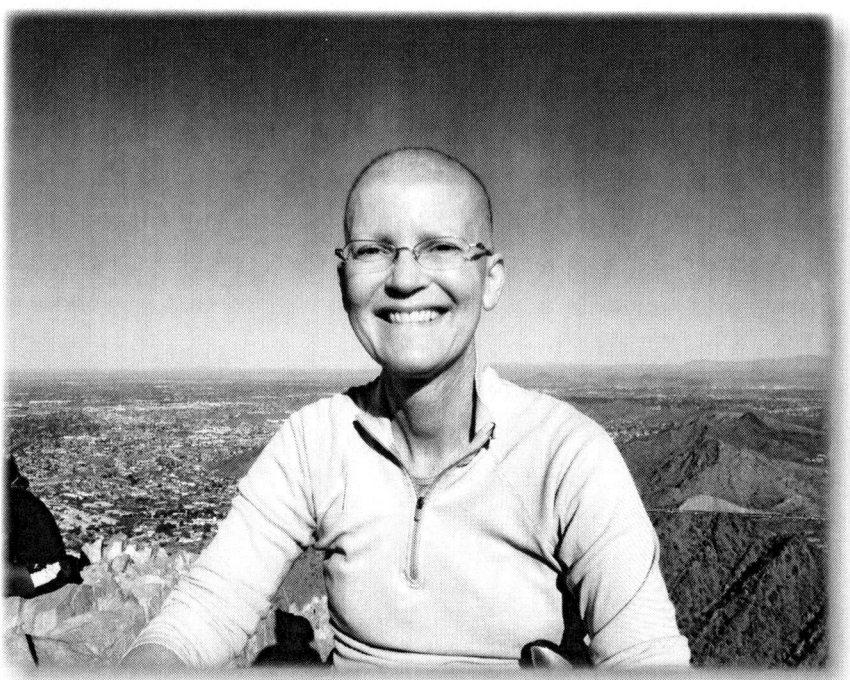

Atop Piestewa Peak today, with new hair sprouting.

On Wednesday, after a few days of letdown and frustration, I talked to three of my doctors and settled on a start date for radiation five weeks after surgery instead of four. The consensus was that a little bit of extra healing time could prevent complications during treatment while posing no risk of a cancer comeback. Phew! I'm glad we got that worked out. It's disconcerting when your physicians give you differing opinions, though apparently it happens all the time.

Early in the week, I was also distressed because fluid seemed to be collecting on the left side of my chest after removal of the drainage tube last Friday. By the time I returned to the plastic surgeon's office on Wednesday morning, I was convinced he would need to insert a needle in my chest to drain the swollen area. To my relief, he said I was simply feeling the tissue expander where my breast used to be. Then he had his assistant inject another 100 ccs of saline into the expander, drawing the skin around it as tight as a newly filled balloon.

Now I know why they call this thing "the rock." When lying on my back, I feel the expander pressing on my chest wall. When bending over or twisting my upper body, I feel its hard edges digging in. Despite the discomfort, I must admit that it creates a breast-like shape I find preferable to a flat space bisected by a scar. I've taken to calling it my "Barbie Boob."

Before I left the plastic surgeon's office, I asked whether I could resume exercising. Three weeks off the trails was making me grumpy. Dr. G. said light cardio exercise would be okay, but no upper-body workouts. "What about hiking?" I asked, not elaborating on the strenuous mountain workouts I enjoy. "Hiking would be fine," he said. At that news, my mood lightened considerably.

On Thursday, three weeks after surgery, I made it three-quarters of the way up Sunrise Peak Trail in northeast Scottsdale, three miles altogether. Today, I climbed all the way to the top of Piestewa Peak on a rocky, rugged stairway of a trail that got my heart thumping. (See photo on previous page.) Not bad after three weeks of slacking. The sun-kissed desert panoramas made me forget all about my aching Barbie Boob.

Prognosis and Prevention

Monday, February 27, 2012

Last Wednesday afternoon, hours after visiting the plastic surgeon, I had another appointment, this one with my medical oncologist. Though chemotherapy ended in late December, I will continue to see Dr. K. long into the future. Where my cancer treatment is concerned, he'll be the one who looks at the big picture and manages my long-term care.

During Wednesday's visit, Moe and I received his assessment of my pathology report. "It would be better if there had been no traces of cancer in the lymph nodes, but it's still a good report," Dr. K. said.

How good? I wondered. Up until now, none of my doctors had provided specifics. Moe must have read my mind. "What are her chances of a recurrence?" he asked.

Estimating likelihood of cancer recurrence is not a perfect science. Factoring in chemo, surgery, radiation, and the impact of estrogen-blocking medications I'll be taking over the next ten years, Dr. K. put my chances of a recurrence between 15 and 20 percent. "Probably closer to 15 percent," he added, explaining that my body type and healthy lifestyle work in my favor.

"That means there's an 80 to 85 percent chance I won't have a recurrence," I said. "That's how we have to look at this."

The doctor smiled. "That's right."

When I asked him what I could do to improve my odds, he advised the following: Limit alcohol to three drinks per week; stay slim (fat cells produce estrogen and my type of breast cancer feeds on estrogen); keep exercising; avoid stress; don't drink out of plastic water bottles with BPA; and don't use antiperspirant with aluminum.

It's nice to know there are a few things in my control that might help prevent the return of this disease. I wish there was more I could do. And maybe there is. Recently, my friend Gayle reminded me that "emotional lifestyle" is perhaps as important to one's health as physical lifestyle.

Do I focus on living well now or worry about getting cancer again? Do I make plans for the future and expect the best-case scenario, or live in fear of that 15 to 20 percent? Do I let uncertainty cast a shadow over my life, or let the sun shine in on my recovery and improving health? Do I talk to family and friends about my sad feelings, or keep them bottled up inside? It's pretty clear which choices are best for my emotional health. I am working hard to adopt attitudes that will help me stay well.

Road Trip!

Saturday, March 3, 2012

A week and a half ago, we decided to postpone the start of my radiation treatments by one week. My doctors agreed that more healing time following surgery would reduce the risk of complications during radiation.

Almost immediately, my husband recognized another benefit of the one-week delay: I could now accompany him on a five-day trip to California for the San Diego Bird Festival. Yes! A Road Trip! And for me, minimal birding required—as long as I didn't mind a stop in Jacumba, a tiny mountain town along the U.S.-Mexico border, to see the tri-colored blackbird.

"No problemo," said I. We've driven past the Jacumba exit on Interstate 8 a few hundred times and I've always wondered about the place. On Thursday evening, my curiosity was satisfied. Only four miles off the highway, Jacumba is an old and not-so-prosperous hamlet within shouting distance of a wall that demarcates the Mexican border.

We rolled into town just before sunset, passing a well-lit market and several lifeless buildings before turning right on (what else?) Jacumba Street. We dodged potholes down a quarter-mile of gravel road and parked next to an embankment. A pair of basset hounds barked at us from a driveway across the street. Moe assured me a pond was located just over the slope, and in it the special blackbirds. With the light fading fast, he grabbed binoculars and spotting scope and dashed up the dirt path.

Reluctantly, I followed him into the cold, windy evening and inadvertently flushed the birds from the reeds in the pond. Because of me, Moe got great looks at the shy red, white, and black flyers he was seeking. Ten minutes later, we were back on the interstate speeding toward San Diego.

As I blog this morning, I am watching through the window of a cozy beachfront condo as surfers hunt for perfect waves near the water's edge. Moe is on a boat nine miles offshore in search of pelagic birds he hasn't seen before—"life birds" he can add to the growing list of North American species he's sighted. A few minutes ago, he texted, GORGEOUS OUT HERE. 2 MORE LIFERS.

Though I'm happy for him, I get seasick just thinking about that boat. I'm delighted to be *by* the water and not *on* it. In a little while, I will walk by the surf, look out over the ocean to the endless horizon, and give thanks for another beautiful day and this much-needed respite from doctors' offices, medical machines, and concerns about my health.

Life's a Beach

Tuesday, March 6, 2012

Five days by the sea is a great cure for what ails you. I walked several miles every day, read books, saw friends, and reconnected with a nephew I hadn't seen in several years. Occasional aches and pains reminded me of what I've been through in recent months, but mostly I forgot about it.

Being a tourist in San Diego is a lot more fun than being a cancer patient in Scottsdale. You get to do things like nosh on seafood kabobs at an oceanfront restaurant while watching the sunset. Or lose yourself in a shopping expedition at convoluted Horton Plaza in San Diego's historic Gaslamp District. You can drive north to La Jolla to watch the sea lions sunning themselves in the rocky cove. Or travel inland a few miles to historic Old Town to dine al fresco on Mexican food and excellent margaritas.

You can also sit on the beach and do nothing but breathe the salt air, listen to the water rushing in and out, and watch the kite surfers rip across the waves. For me, the beach has intangible healing properties and no unpleasant side effects, as long as you apply sunscreen.

We awoke this morning to a cool and cloudy day, weather that made it easier to pack up the car and head home to Arizona.

Beating Back "The Monster"

Sunday, March 11, 2012

In the first month after my breast cancer diagnosis, I was sometimes overwhelmed by the fear of dying. I touched on this in a blog post last year titled, "The Silver Lining" (September 17, 2011).

Fear of death, also known as "The Monster," has shadowed me since August, stepping out of the darkness to terrorize me when I have been most vulnerable. When the fire of my spirit burns bright, stoked by courage, hope, faith, determination, and the support and encouragement of loved ones, The Monster doesn't stand a chance. He slinks into the deep recesses of my psyche and waits for doubt, discouragement, weariness, and self-pity to dampen my spirit and dim my flame.

Anyone who has faced a life-threatening disease has battled The Monster. He arrives to spew gloom and doom from his hideous mouth when you are at your lowest. "Imagine a world in which you are not present," he hisses into your ear. "Don't get up, don't get dressed, and don't make plans, because you are going to die."

The Monster will take you to the pits of despair, if you let him. When he comes calling, I have learned to play the "opposite game." I imagine watching my children graduate from college. I picture myself with grandchildren on my lap. I see a very old woman, the future me, walking hand-in-hand with an even older man, the future Moe. I get up, get going, make plans, keep living. I am optimistic. I am fearless. My inner fire rages. The Monster is no match for me. I picture him in full retreat, along with my cancer.

As a friend pointed out to me last fall, "You may walk through the Valley of the Shadow of Death, but it is still only 'IN THE SHADOW OF.'"

Postscript: The above post generated a lot of feedback, perhaps because everyone can relate to the fear of death on some level. My words seemed to resonate most strongly with a breast cancer survivor who commented, "You nailed this one…. I imagined myself as a generation older, with a short gray ponytail. Funny how we are averse to aging when life is just status quo, but embrace it when we realize it is a goal."

I still grapple with The Monster, usually when I visit the doctor for check-ups or hear about another cancer survivor who's had a recurrence. Sometimes when I am making plans, an icy voice whispers from the dark recesses of my psyche, "If you're still here by then…." I shiver a little, but go ahead with my life and hope that someday The Monster will be silenced.

RADIATION

"Courage doesn't always roar. Sometimes courage is the quiet voice at the end of the day saying, 'I will try again tomorrow.'"

—Mary Anne Radmacher

Heads or Tails?

Tuesday, March 13, 2012

A few years ago, an uncle of mine received radiation for prostate cancer. He was instructed to come to the medical building for his treatment at the same time every day for several weeks. One day, while he was on the table being bombarded with invisible radioactive beams, he realized that something was wrong. The radiation machine seemed to be targeting his head instead of his nether regions.

At first he couldn't make heads or tails of the situation (sorry, couldn't resist!), but eventually his radiation technicians admitted they had mistaken him for another patient and irradiated his brain. This only happened once, and seemed to do my uncle no harm, though he did have to endure some ribbing from the family. Until now, I couldn't imagine how such a blatant mistake might have happened. On Friday, I went to Suite 101 in Piper Cancer Center and had my first encounter with a radiation machine. Not all of these devices are the same, but the one administering my treatments looks like a miniature flying saucer attached to a large metal arm. It is a two-foot-wide, six-inch-thick metal disc with a foot-wide square of glass at its center. Behind the glass, thin metal strips move sideways to create openings in programmed patterns that shape the way radiation is sent into a patient's body.

As I observed the machine for the first time, it seemed completely mysterious. For all I could tell, the flying saucer might have been shooting beams at my ear, chin, chest, or belly button. I quickly developed a more sympathetic view of my uncle's predicament.

Friday's visit was not for treatment, but to make locational markings in Sharpie on the geography of my chest and to take "films" (actually crude x-rays) to make sure things (such as the tissue expander) underneath my skin had not changed position. As I lay on the table with my arms over my head, my hands gripping pegs, four people stood over me holding tiny rulers next to various points around my Barbie Boob. They slid me around until the Sharpie Xs on my chest lined up with the red lines of light that shone down from overhead. Then they left the room while the machine took radiation-based pictures.

I felt like the human in a sci-fi movie that has been captured by aliens and taken onto their strange ship for closer examination. When they were done, I was released unharmed and told to return on Monday for my first treatment.

The space people seem to know what they're doing. Monday's visit was painless and relatively quick. I got on the table, reached my arms overhead to grasp the pegs, and let them move me into the proper position. After they left the room, the flying saucer moved in an arc over my torso, stopping at various angles and locations to send cancer-killing radiation into my chest and armpit on the left side. Meanwhile, I was entertained by a musical accompaniment of short clicks and long beeps. A computer in the next room coordinated the whole operation. Fifteen minutes later, I was free to go.

I will have close encounters with the strange machine every Monday through Friday for the next six-and-a-half weeks. During today's visit, I determined that the technicians are not space people after all. When I told the one called Keith that I was going to a Major League spring training game this afternoon, he proudly showed me his bobble head doll of Diamondbacks Manager Kirk Gibson. Turns out Keith lived in Detroit when Gibson played for the Tigers.

One Week Down, 5½ to Go

Friday, March 16, 2012

I'm hoping each week of radiation passes as quickly as this one. I went in every day, Monday through Friday, for a fifteen-minute treatment. Though the radioactive particles bombarding my body were invisible, I quickly felt their effects. On the way home from my first treatment on Monday, a mild burning/chafing sensation began on the rim of my armpit and across the top of my Barbie Boob. The discomfort increased after Tuesday's treatment.

On Wednesday, I had my weekly consultation with the radiation oncologist, who gave me samples of Andra Sina Emerald Aloe Relief Lotion. This feel-good cream is soothing my sore areas. After five treatments, my radiated skin is tight and tender, but not unbearably so. I'm hoping the lotion will stop the formation of stretch marks that may be developing along Barbie's midsection.

Dr. T. showed me computer models of my chest that she used to develop my radiation treatment plan. Pictured on the monitor were my expander implant, heart, lung, and other important areas outlined in different colors. The doctor said the plan she created should minimize spillover radiation to my heart and left lung as much as possible, "because I know you are an active person." Still, there will be some spillover and some mild damage to these vital organs.

When I asked whether the damage would be repaired over time, she said yes. Then Dr. T. told me about a former patient who ran a marathon a year or so after treatment. "She inspired me to run my first half-marathon," the doctor said.

That conversation was tremendously reassuring. I have been out on three hikes and a long walk in the park this week, far from my peak performance levels though plugging along at a steady pace. I look forward to regaining my former fitness level sometime in the future.

For now, my goal is simply to keep exercising throughout the six-and-a-half weeks of fatigue-inducing radiation.

A Way Up the Mountain

Tuesday, March 20, 2012

Since I got clearance to resume hiking, almost four weeks ago, I have been on the slopes of all my favorite local peaks except one, Camelback Mountain. As I'm sure I've mentioned before, the Echo Canyon Trail up Camelback is extremely rugged and strenuous. Along a few of the steepest stretches, railings constructed of metal piping help hikers keep their purchase on the rock.

Prior to my mastectomy, I hiked Echo Canyon Trail with friends about once a week. Now, I'm afraid I lack the strength in my left arm to hold onto those pipes or do much climbing. I need to build myself up and get through radiation before I try it again. Last week, while I was thinking about how much I've missed hiking Camelback and the view from the top, an obvious solution presented itself. There is another path up Camelback, the Cholla Trail. While still challenging and a bit longer than Echo, it is not quite as difficult.

Today, my hiking buddies and I made our way up the Cholla Trail under blue skies and temperatures in the 60s. It was a perfect hiking day, and unusually cool for late March in Phoenix. I stood atop the peak with Pam, Angie, and Barclay, looking west toward the downtown skyline, and thought, *So good to be back.*

A few hours later, I bounced into Piper Cancer Center for radiation and my weekly visit with the radiation oncologist. She said it was okay to start exercises for my left arm and recommended yoga to help with flexibility. "After chemo, surgery and radiation, you have a different, more fragile body," she added. "You need to be careful with it, avoiding extreme hot and cold temperatures, for example."

Always one to push the boundaries of my limitations, I didn't like hearing that. How do you avoid extreme heat while hiking in Phoenix during the summer? Impossible. But a smart hiker will proceed with caution, listening to her body and slowing down when necessary. That will be my approach. One way or another, I will find a way up the mountain.

Hair!

Thursday, March 22, 2012

> *Hair, hair, hair, hair, hair, hair, hair*
> *Flow it, show it*
> *Long as God can grow it*
> *My hair*

> Can't yet flow it, still want to show it
> Three months after chemo
> My hair

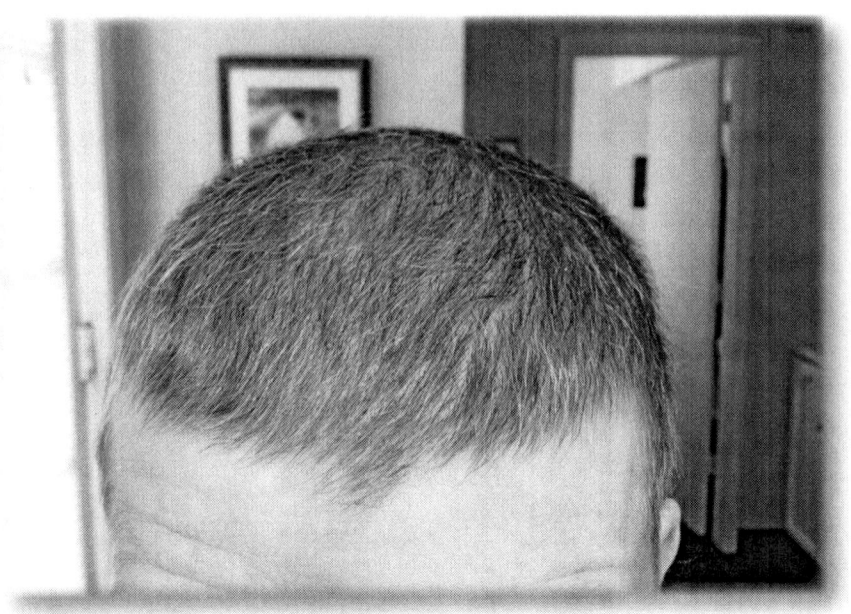

I want it long, straight, curly, fuzzy
Snaggy, shaggy, ratty, matty
Oily, greasy, fleecy
Shining, gleaming, streaming
Flaxen, waxen....

Hair, hair, hair, hair, hair, hair, hair
Spiky, swirly, not too girly
Too short to be twirly
My hair

Radiation

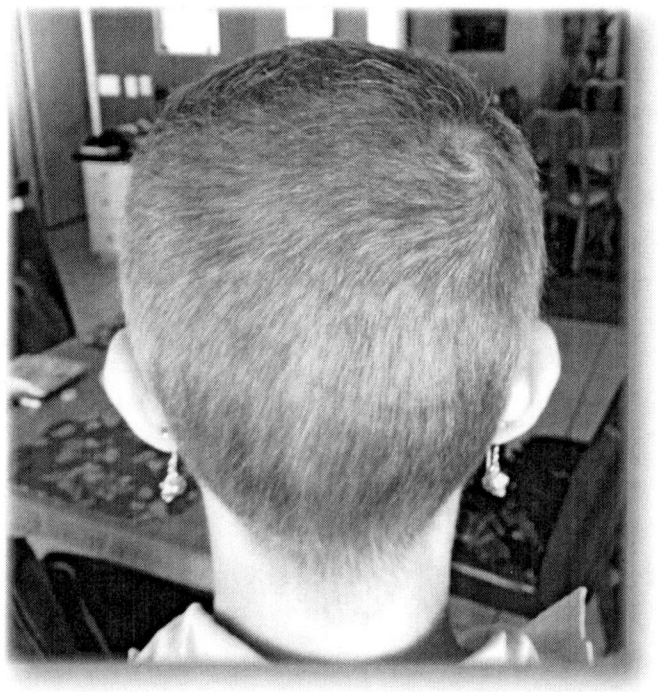

A home for fleas
A hive for bees
A nest for birds
There ain't no words
For the beauty, the splendor, the wonder
Of my hair

Graying but staying
There is no more delaying
And finally I am getting some
HAIR, HAIR, HAIR, HAIR, HAIR, HAIR, HAIR!

(Lyrics in italics by Gerome Ragni from the musical *Hair*, 1967.)

Postscript: The return of my hair brought exhilaration. It was like my body saying, "Your time in Chemoworld is over. Welcome back to the land of the living." I wasn't sure what color or texture my new hair would take on, but I was all set to love it. One of my doctors said all of her patients had gray, kinky locks following chemo. I would have accepted that, but my mane grew in dark, thick, and curly, and has morphed over time back into its pre-cancer waviness. The gray strands are few and far between.

Radiation: A Nice Place to Visit, but I Wouldn't Want to Live There

Tuesday, March 27, 2012

Yesterday brought my eleventh radiation treatment out of thirty-three. "You're one-third of the way through and doing great," Moe said as he hugged me.

I have established a very satisfying Monday through Friday routine: Hike with friends in the morning (a particularly mood-enhancing activity during our gorgeous spring weather), go for radiation in the afternoon, and spend the rest of my time doing normal things like housework, grocery shopping, cooking, reading, and writing. Fatigue creeps up on me late in the day, but so far hasn't been too bad.

Today at 1:15, I will go for my next treatment. Linda, the receptionist, will greet me by name and offer a welcoming smile. Within a few minutes of my arrival, Keith or Joe will come to the waiting room to lead me back to the machine. Roxy might be there, too. They'll help me onto the table, where I will unbutton my shirt and raise my arms over my head so they can align the Xs on my chest with the red laser lines from overhead. Then they will leave the room, and I will lie there until the mini-spaceship device is done sending radioactive beams into my body. Who can complain about 10–15 minutes of relaxation in a dimly lit room?

My brain uses that time to browse its data banks for happy thoughts. The pleasure of this morning's hike, for example, or the look on my daughter's face last Friday when she received the "large envelope" from Occidental College (her parents' alma mater) welcoming her to the class of 2016. On the way out of radiation, I will say "Hi" to Joyce, a nurse and hiking enthusiast who treks into the Grand Canyon every April. We've already shared several stories of our adventures there.

On Tuesdays, I also have my weekly visit with the radiation oncologist, Dr. T. Born in Burma, she immigrated to the United States as a girl and worked very hard to learn English and do well enough in school to become a doctor. Despite many obstacles, she made her American dream come true.

I'm not thrilled that I have to undergo radiation, but I'm glad it's in this place with these people.

Lessons from the Cabin

Monday, April 2, 2012

Twenty-two years ago this June, when I was pregnant with Brian, Moe read a newspaper article about a terrible fire that burned thousands of acres of forest north of Payson, Arizona. A crew of convicts on work furlough died fighting the "Dude Fire." We didn't know it at the time, but this was the first of several major forest fires to plague our drought-stricken state over the next twenty years.

After reading aloud excerpts from the article, Moe said, "This may sound crazy, but there will never be a better time to buy land up there." It *did* sound crazy. While he was dreaming of a property

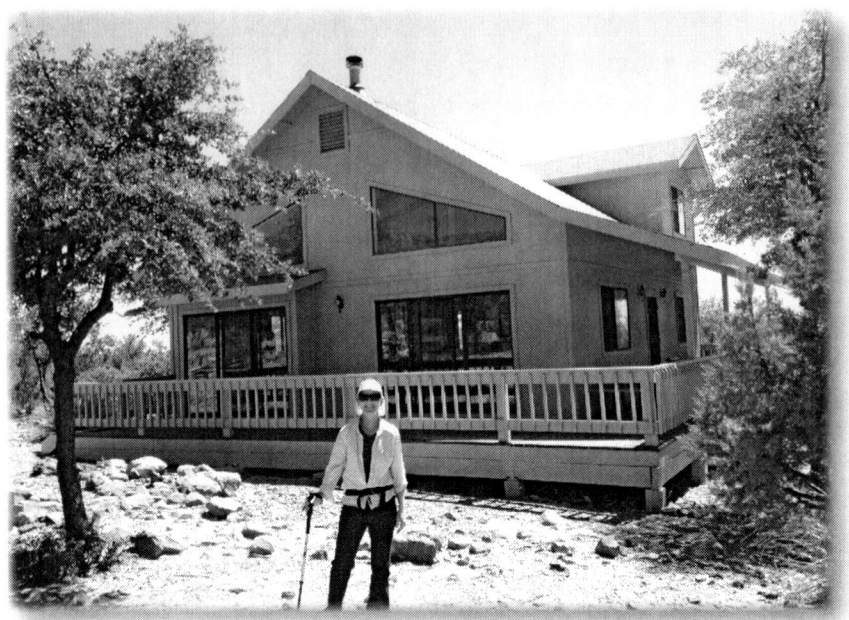

Bell cabin north of Payson, Arizona.

in the high country, I was poring over *What to Expect While You're Expecting* and trying to contain my anxiety over the impending birth of our first child. Still, I could see his point. We agreed we'd drive up there and take a look around after the baby was born.

That fall, when Brian was six weeks old, we finally made the ninety-mile trip to Bonita Creek. Prior to being caught in the crosshairs of the Dude Fire, it had been a hamlet of cabins and small homes set within tall pines at an elevation of 6,000 feet. Located at the base of the Mogollon Rim, a thousand-foot up-thrust of land that lets you know you are entering northern Arizona, Bonita Creek boasted a four-season climate and proximity to Phoenix that made it ideal for weekend getaways.

We were eager to see for ourselves what the area looked like after the fire. It wasn't pretty. In some places, the Ponderosa pine forest had been burned into oblivion; in others, charred standing tree trunks and their fallen brothers populated an ash-covered landscape.

Amid the devastation, we also saw unobstructed views of the rim to the north and rolling foothills to the south. Downhill from the high street, we discovered a flowing stream lined with many tall pines that had escaped the flames. The community was a wreck from the fire, but it had potential.

We could build a cabin with a view there, and take hikes along the pretty creek. Half-acre lots with septic tanks could be purchased for a song. The question was, how long until Mother Nature worked her magic and made a new forest begin to rise out of the ashes? How long until we could go for a walk and not get soot on our clothes?

No one could tell us, exactly. We took a chance (the price was right) and bought a view lot on the high street. Three years later, when grass, manzanita, oak, and juniper began to reappear, we decided to build.

Our place at Bonita Creek has been a refuge for us ever since. A place away from TV and technology when the kids were growing up. A place close to nature but offering a bath at the end of the day. A place to observe wildlife—including elk, deer, woodpeckers, hawks, jays, hummingbirds, and raccoons—and view the Milky Way from our back deck. A place for Moe to chop wood and forget work stress, and for me to read, write, and recover from medical treatments during my cancer journey.

This past weekend, Moe and I noticed that the trees around the cabin have grown so tall that they are starting to obstruct our views. Terrain once burned into a blackened wasteland is now home to a thriving oak forest with Ponderosa pines sprinkled here and there. Bonita Creek's recovery over two decades is a testament to nature's resiliency.

Watching the jays flit in and out of the twenty-foot-tall oak towering over our rock driveway, I thought about how landscapes, plants, animals, and even humans are capable of bouncing back from terrible ravages. We are designed to endure, recover, survive, and thrive.

With a lot of help from modern medicine, this process is happening inside my body right now. I see it in the return of my hair, appetite, physical strength, sense of humor, and zest for life. Like the area around our cabin, I have been scarred and forever changed, but also reborn.

"I'm Not Tired!"

Saturday, April 7, 2012

Like a grumpy three-year-old before naptime, I keep insisting, "I'm not tired!" It's not true, of course. After four weeks of radiation, fatigue is present during most of my waking hours. I'm also having a harder time hiking up the steepest sections of my favorite mountain trails.

Last Tuesday, on the "easy" side of Camelback Mountain, I struggled up a steep pitch and had to sit down. I looked at the top of the peak and shook my head. "I don't think I'm going to make it today," I told my hiking companion. I sent her on to the summit and made myself comfortable on a chair-sized rock.

After a few minutes, my breathing returned to normal and I stopped feeling light-headed. *Maybe I can go a little farther,* I thought, getting to my feet. Slowly but steadily, I made my way across the craggy ridge and up the last rocky slope to the top. With metropolitan Phoenix stretched out below me, I caught my breath and reflected on what I had learned about tiredness, just then and in recent weeks.

Fatigue is not an insurmountable obstacle. When it's mild, you can push through it. When it's kicking your butt on the hiking trail, a few minutes of rest can conquer it. Listen to your body, slow down if you have to, rest when you must, but keep on going. You might be surprised what you can accomplish.

Tour de California

Thursday, April 12, 2012

I drove my best friend to the airport yesterday. He flew to Sacramento, California to embark on an 800-mile bicycle ride from the California capital south to San Diego. Along the way, he will hug road shoulders and bike lanes through Napa Valley, San Francisco, Los Angeles, and many points in between. He'll have a flashing light on the back of his bike and will wear a florescent yellow jersey that glows like a lighthouse beacon. I hope it's enough to make him visible to clueless drivers.

As readers may recall, Moe had a collision with a shopping cart a few months ago that banged him up but did no permanent damage. A week later, he was back in the saddle, having replaced a broken front wheel on his bike, and ignoring the pain of a cracked rib. Some people might have asked their spouses to quit cycling after such an accident, but I knew that would only make my adventuresome husband miserable. In the past several months, he has pedaled away a lot of his stress over my breast cancer treatment. So, instead of asking him to quit, I encouraged him to buy a new and better bike. He did, and he kept training for this ride.

Moe's college and medical school buddy Bob O., with whom he rode 400 miles across Arizona last year, invited Moe on the California trek. Almost three years ago, Bob's son Eric was killed on his bicycle by a young woman suspected of texting while driving. Bob now cycles to raise awareness about the dangers of distracted driving. Last year, he pedaled from his home state of California to Florida, stopping to speak at high schools and state houses. His message is printed on the back of his cycling jersey: "Please drive cell free." This year's ride aims to promote stiffer penalties for distracted driving in California.

Moe, Bob, and three or four others in their small group expect to cycle seventy to eighty miles a day for the next eleven days. They began their journey this morning in Sacramento, probably in the rain, though I haven't heard yet. I wish them smooth (and mostly dry) pavement, wide bike lanes, only distant encounters with alert and courteous drivers, plenty of cold beer and hearty food at the end of each day, and a soft bed to collapse into. Radiation seems tame by comparison.

What's New: Radiation and Tour de California

Sunday, April 15, 2012

On Friday, I completed my fifth week of radiation. I arrived early so the medical team could make preparations to "boost" the dose to the scar that cuts across the top of my Barbie Boob. Sharpie in hand, the radiation oncologist drew a dotted line around the scar, and then the technicians took "films" and digital pictures.

They were creating a template from which a block will be made with a cutout, targeting Barbie's scar. The block will be attached to the radiation machine as part of my last eight treatments. Breast cancer often recurs along mastectomy scars, where skin overlaps to close up the wound. My doctor wants to be sure this area receives enough rays to kill any unseen cancer cells.

Two-and-a-half months after surgery, the scar is well healed. I feel confident that it will withstand the boost in radiation dose. Five weeks of therapy has given the skin on my left chest and armpit a sunburned appearance. This skin seems fragile, but only bothers me when something rough brushes against it. In a week and a half, I will put the sunburn and fatigue of radiation behind me. I can't wait to celebrate the end of treatment on April 25.

Tour de California update: After four days and more than 300 miles of travel on his bike, Moe is tired but content. Day one, Sacramento to Napa, he and his buds rode through rain and up a mountain. Day two, Napa to San Francisco, they enjoyed clear weather and a glorious view of the Golden Gate Bridge. Day three, San Francisco to Santa Cruz, they pedaled past Half Moon Bay, alternating between rolling hills and coastline. Day four (today), they traveled a challenging 100 miles from Santa Cruz to King City. No major mishaps so far, though Moe did confess that a bus passed within a foot of him on the road yesterday, and a bee flew into his helmet today and dropped down into his jersey and stung him on the chest. "It hurt like hell," he said, "but Bob pulled out the stinger and we rode on."

Last Days of Radiation

Friday, April 20, 2012

Since Tuesday, my radiation treatment has focused on the scar along the top of my fake breast, where skin spared during my mastectomy meets and overlaps. Rays shoot from the radiation machine to the scar through a cutout in a block of radiation-stopping materials. This metal block, attached to the machine with a bracket, was custom-made just for me.

The whole apparatus is remotely controlled to within an inch or two of the scar, but first a technician places a rectangle of quarter-inch thick gel over Barbie. Apparently, the gel acts like extra layers of skin, and prevents the radiation from penetrating too deeply beneath the scar.

I observe the block, the gel, the machine that looks like a mini-spaceship, and the people hovering over me, and think about all the medical resources and personnel that have been directed toward eradicating my breast cancer during the past eight months: ultra-sounds, biopsies, and MRIs; three powerful chemo drugs, a host of anti-nausea drugs, countless blood tests, and shots to boost my white count; a port implanted in my chest to receive chemo, surgery to remove my breast, and a tissue expander put in its place to make me look and feel normal.

Radiologists, pathologists, oncologists, surgeons, chemo nurses, surgical staff, the radiation team, and many others have rallied to my side.

The costs have been astronomical. We have good insurance, but it's shocking when you find out the shot you need after chemo has a $700 price tag, or that insurance doesn't cover a $3,000 genetic test that your doctor recommends. When all is said and done, the total cost of my treatment will be well into six figures. What is the value of one human life? I don't know, but I'm grateful for the efforts and resources that have been devoted to saving mine.

These are some of the things I'm thinking about in the last days of radiation. One moment, I am elated that the treatment phase of this experience (chemo, surgery, and radiation) is almost over; the next moment, emotions rise up that I can't begin to explain. In many respects, fighting breast cancer has been like my most challenging mountain climb, up Montana's Granite Peak. Along the way, we crossed raging streams, bushwhacked our way up overgrown trails, carried sixty-pound packs across mile-long boulder fields, crossed steep slopes of loose talus, trod carefully over snowfields and glacier, and finally rock climbed our way to the top.

It took everything I had to reach the top of that mountain. I over-came exhaustion, fear, anger, hunger, and thirst. At the summit, I collapsed on the rocks and let out a sob of relief. I suspect I may have a similar reaction at the end of radiation.

My Iron Man

Monday, April 23, 2012

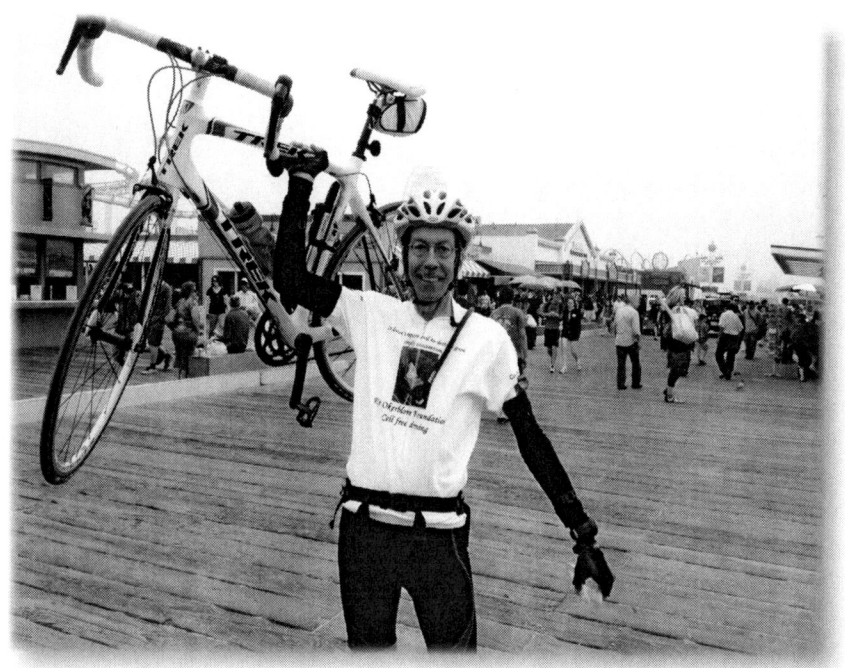

Moe, shown above at Santa Monica Pier, returned home from his epic bike ride last night. He rode 706 miles on the route from Sacramento to San Diego. The smile on his face says it all. It's been great to have an iron man by my side during breast cancer treatment.

Crossing the Finish Line

Wednesday, April 25, 2012

During much of the past eight months, the last day of treatment seemed like a distant dream. Eight chemo infusions over four months was

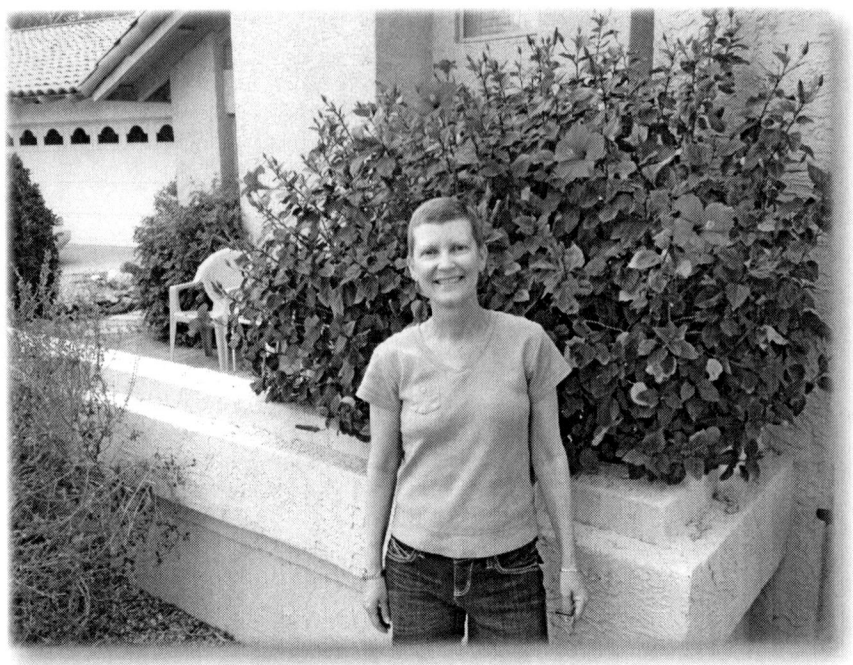

forever. Nausea, a bad taste in the mouth, bone pain, muscle aches, exhaustion. It took all my available energy to get through that, much less think about what came next. Surgery and its aftermath were all-consuming as well. Pains, drains, forced inactivity, dark thoughts creeping in. Then came radiation, a daily meeting with the machine that dispensed cancer-killing, fatigue-inducing invisible rays. Thirty-three treatments over six-and-a-half weeks. It seemed like it would never be over, but today it is.

I am done with the major elements of breast cancer treatment. I got through it the only way I could, one step at a time. Some of those strides were physical, along the hiking trail, while others were mental, carrying me through each challenge in the present moment. By staying in the "now," I avoided becoming overwhelmed by the daunting and lengthy treatment plan. When you are able to hike up Camelback Mountain on your last day of treatment, as I did this morning, you know things have gone just about as smoothly as possible.

To borrow a metaphor from Hillary Clinton, it took a village to bring me to the mountaintop this morning. My village included dedicated health care providers and the best friends and family anyone could hope for. My village took care of me and loved me through this. If not for breast cancer, I might never have known the depth of their love. If I start to forget, I have a box full of greeting cards, countless gifts, and a cabinet overflowing with plastic containers from meals delivered during chemo to remind me.

I pray I'll never have to go through breast cancer treatment again, but I don't want to live in fear of that possibility. I choose to celebrate today and appreciate every good thing and person in my life. I choose to embrace the future with optimism and enthusiasm. I look forward to the return of my full strength and stamina, which will come in handy as I hike rim-to-rim across the Grand Canyon in October.

Tomorrow I transition to the post-treatment stage of my breast cancer experience, which will involve estrogen-blocking pills; a cancer-prevention lifestyle; ongoing tests and doctor visits; and sometime next winter, the completion of breast reconstruction. But first things first, tonight we celebrate!

Postscript: It wasn't a fancy celebration. We ordered takeout from our favorite Thai restaurant, and then Moe, Brian, Emily, and I ate together at the kitchen table. I just wanted to share my relief—and joy—with those I loved most. No amount of fine food or drink could have provided more of a high than the one I was already feeling. The smile in the previous photo was from the inside out because, I MADE IT!

You might think it would have been an emotional evening, but it wasn't. After eight months on the cancer roller coaster, my family was more than ready for the ride to be over. They offered high-fives rather than tearful congratulations, and that was fine with me. Sometimes it takes a while for emotions to catch up with events in our lives.

5 RECOVERY

"Happiness is not something you postpone for the future; it is something you design for the present."
—Jim Rohn

Gifts of Yoga

Tuesday, May 1, 2012

Until recently, I viewed yoga in the 2000s much the same way as I saw aerobics in the 1980s—a trendy activity with some health benefits, but not a good fit for me. At the urging of my yoga-loving friends and one of my doctors, I decided to give the posing pursuit another chance.

Two weeks ago I drove thirty minutes across town to go with my friend Gayle to a yoga studio near her house. Gayle had invited me to take a class with one of her favorite instructors, a breast cancer survivor. Sally Jo began her class by encouraging everyone to focus on "just this," meaning the present moment. She talked about how hard it can be to stay mentally where you are, and not leap ahead. Unfamiliar with the yoga moves, I had no trouble keeping my mind on "just this," but I appreciated the message. How often have I let my attention stray to the next item on my agenda, rather than being fully engaged in the now?

Sally Jo's class wasn't easy for me. My hiker's body is not very flexible, especially after cancer treatment. Sitting on a mat with my back straight and legs crossed felt unnatural, as did most of the poses. I listened to Sally Jo's instructions, breathing in and out with the movements, and my discomfort eased. "Warrior," "sun salutation," "downward dog"—I did these poses and others to the best of my limited ability. In yoga, I learned, whatever you can do is good enough.

After an hour and a half of mindful movement, we lay on our mats with our eyes closed for several minutes. When we got up, my body felt completely relaxed. No kinks or stiffness anywhere. My mental kinks had disappeared as well. I had come to yoga to work on flexibility and upper-body strength, but discovered something more.

Sally Jo told me not to worry about the limited range of motion in my left arm. Swinging around her arm on the side where she'd had a mastectomy and full dissection of the lymph nodes in her armpit, she said, "It will all come back, just like this."

That first class with Gayle and Sally Jo gave me the confidence to try yoga at the cancer center five minutes from my house. The classes there are free for life to cancer survivors. Each teacher proceeds in her own way, but always with an emphasis on breathing through the movements and staying focused on the present moment. For me, the result has been the same at the end of every class: a relaxed body and a calm mind. Studies have shown that yoga is good for breast cancer patients and survivors. Now I know why.

"Let go of past regrets and future worries," one instructor encouraged. "Live in gratitude, joy, and peace." That might be the best advice I've ever heard.

I went to yoga with Gayle again yesterday. We had tea afterward, and I told her that I hadn't really understood yoga or had the patience for it in the past. "I wasn't ready for it until now," I said. She just nodded and smiled.

Sorting Out the Costs of Cancer Treatment

Monday, May 7, 2012

When I finished the acute phase of breast cancer treatment, I wanted to know what it all cost. My husband, who might have been an accountant if medicine hadn't captured his fancy, crunched some numbers for me. Medical billing is a mysterious science. For each doctor visit, procedure, or treatment, we received a bill with three amounts listed: the total charges, the amount insurance would pay, and how much we owed. In an earlier post, I estimated that costs would reach well into six figures. Turns out I was right.

Total charges for chemo, surgery, and radiation, including scans, lab work, shots, and co-pays for doctor visits: $283,015. Amount paid by insurance: $103,658. Amount we've paid: $13,012. To break things down further, radiation made up roughly 41 percent of the total charges, chemo 34 percent, and surgery 25 percent.

You don't have to be a math whiz to see that there's a big difference between total medical charges and the amounts paid by insurance and the consumer. If you have insurance, this difference is forgiven. If you don't have insurance, you have to pay the full amount or try to negotiate better terms with your care providers.

In any case, fighting cancer is an expensive proposition. The costs could easily bankrupt an average family without insurance. I'm grateful I didn't have to worry about whether I could afford treatment while battling a life-threatening disease. I wish no one did.

The Pill (no, not that one)

Thursday, May 10, 2012

After two glorious weeks devoid of medical treatments and medication, I took a pill with breakfast this morning. My oncologist says I'll have to keep this habit for the next ten years. The round white tablet called Tamoxifen is an estrogen-blocking drug. My type of breast cancer thrives on estrogen the way a plant flourishes on Miracle-Gro. Reducing estrogen in my body greatly lowers my chance of a recurrence, a compelling reason to start popping a pill every day.

"Almost everyone on Tamoxifen gets hot flashes," the doctor said as he gave me the prescription. "One in a thousand gets blood clots, so don't ignore any persistent pain in your calves. One in two thousand gets uterine cancer, but that's very treatable."

Holy sh––! I thought as he described this good news/bad news drug. Friends had told me about other side effects, including mouth sores and weight gain. I had noticed that Tamoxifen is prescribed in the same 20 mg dose for everyone, which gave me an idea. "Could I take a lower dose, since I am smaller than most women?" I asked.

"No," he replied firmly, leaving me to assume that the drug has not been proven effective in lower doses. Oh well.

This morning I reminded myself that none of Tamoxifen's side effects would be as bad as a return of my cancer. I swallowed the pill and got on with my day.

Postscript: The doctor was right—hot flashes have been a fixture of my life since starting Tamoxifen. While "flashing" on an already hot Arizona day, I try to bear it without complaint, because more than any other preventive measure, that little white pill may be what keeps me cancer free.

Vegas!

Thursday, May 17, 2012

There's nothing like the tang of a mimosa on your tongue as you head to the airport for a flight to Las Vegas. My three hiking pals

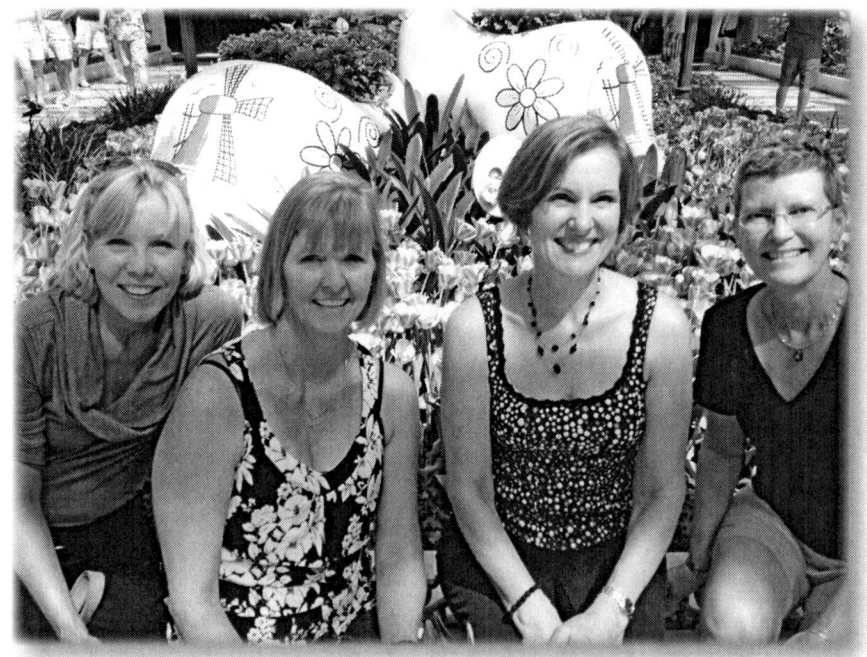

Barclay, Angie, Pam and me by the indoor gardens at Bellagio.

and I agreed on this point after we clinked our champagne flutes and toasted Pam's birthday, the end of my treatment, and the kickoff to a memorable Mother's Day weekend for all of us.

From last Friday morning to Saturday night, we were four moms in Sin City. Four non-gamblers in to see a Cirque du Soleil show, have a few good meals, hang out by the musical fountain at Bellagio, do a little shopping, and go home with smiles on our faces.

"Ka," the Cirque du Soleil show we saw at the MGM Grand, was mesmerizing. Within a loose storyline of twins separated by warfare, there were shipwrecks, clowns, acrobats, dancers, trapeze artists, and a baton twirler better than any you've ever seen on the 50-yard line. Somehow it all hung together and had us shaking our heads in amazement at the end.

Early on in our thirty-hour adventure, I told the girls my 99-cent shrimp story, the perfect metaphor for Las Vegas. In the 1980s, when Moe and I were visiting "Lost Wages" with friends, a large sign along the Strip caught our eye. "Shrimp Cocktail, 99 cents," it said. We piled into the restaurant in front of the sign, mouths watering in anticipation.

Soon after placing our order, we received ice-packed goblets draped with jumbo shrimp so luscious you'd swear they did time in the gym. "Jackpot!" we all thought, until the bill arrived. Somewhere between the sign and our seats at the counter, the 99-cent shrimp cocktails had morphed into ten-dollar apiece delicacies.

"Excuse me Miss, but the sign outside says 'Shrimp Cocktail, 99 cents,'" someone said to the waitress.

"Oh, that's for the place next door," she said, pointing to the take-out window of a shack in the shadow of her restaurant. I learned some valuable lessons that day. In Las Vegas, things often are not what they seem. And if something seems too good to be true, it usually is.

Like "Ka," Las Vegas is a fantasy world that can dazzle and captivate. It's a fun place to escape to for a little while, but stay too long and its charms wear off. We four moms could have done without the pole dancer on the casino floor at the MGM Grand, creepy men on the sidewalks dispensing discount coupons to adult shows, and the way casino designers make it nearly impossible to find an exit to the outdoors.

When we spotted a bright red Audi sport sedan perched atop a bank of slot machines at the MGM, we were tempted to put some coins in the slots. The impulse didn't last long. We were about as likely to win that sweet ride as to find a 99-cent shrimp cocktail in 2012 Las Vegas. We spent our money on clothes and shoes instead.

Like Cinderella climbing into her carriage before midnight, Angie, Pam, Barclay, and I boarded our plane back to Phoenix on

Saturday night more charmed than jaded. For a day-and-a-half, none of us cleaned house, prepared meals, ferried kids to activities, broke up sibling squabbles, or thought about recent life-threatening illnesses. Thanks to Las Vegas, we were all a little bit more "chill" on Mother's Day this year.

The Sisterhood

Friday, May 18, 2012

A few days ago, hot and exhausted after hiking and running errands in 100-degree heat, I sought respite at the yogurt shop. While sprinkling dark chocolate chips over my cup of blood red orange sorbet, I overheard the customer ahead of me thanking the shop owner for her sweet treat.

"I'll see you again in two weeks, after my next chemo," she said.

At her mention of chemo I looked up. The woman was wearing a pink ball cap over her shorn head.

"I had chemo for breast cancer at the end of last year," I said. "What kind of cancer do you have?"

"My two sisters and I were on the *Today* show recently," she said. "We've all been fighting breast cancer at the same time."

Her name was Kathleen "Sunshine" O'Brien. Her mother had died of breast cancer, and she and her sisters recently learned that they carry the BRCA2 gene. In the past year-and-a-half, two of the O'Briens had been diagnosed with Stage 3 disease and the other with Stage 2.

"After the *Today* segment, we were contacted by two other sets of O'Brien sisters who've also battled breast cancer," Sunshine added. "There is a whole sisterhood of women like us."

She held out her arm and shook a bracelet loaded with breast cancer-related silver charms. "This was sent to me from a woman in Texas," she said. "A survivor gave it to her when she was having treatment, and now she's passed it on to me."

I wrote down my blog link for Kathleen, and she gave me a business card with a picture of the three O'Brien sisters. A logo above them features three pink ribbons and the words "3 Sisters Survival." Each woman wears a white T-shirt with two red circles and a slash over the words "breast cancer" where their breasts used to be. "That's me on the left," she said, pointing to herself with long blond hair. The look on her face told me just how much she wished to look like her old self again.

I left the yogurt shop marveling at the prevalence of breast cancer among American women (about 1 in 8 will get it), and also at how we gain strength from one another. One of my good friends had a mastectomy a week ago. She helped me stay focused on the positive during my cancer treatment, and now it's my turn to support her. That's how things are in our sisterhood. We pass on advice, lucky charms, love, encouragement, and whatever else we can to new members of this growing club none of us chose to join.

The End Is the Beginning

Saturday, May 26, 2012

Last Tuesday, Moe, Brian, and I attended Emily's high school graduation in an air-conditioned sports arena at Arizona State University. Our girl was seated in the front row on the arena floor, a place of honor for a select group from her class. She was recognized for being in the Top 5 percent, a National Merit Commended Scholar, and the Scottsdale Charros Outstanding Female Senior from Chaparral High School. Looking down at her from the stands, it was hard to stop smiling. Moe and I were proud of her accomplishments, of course, but

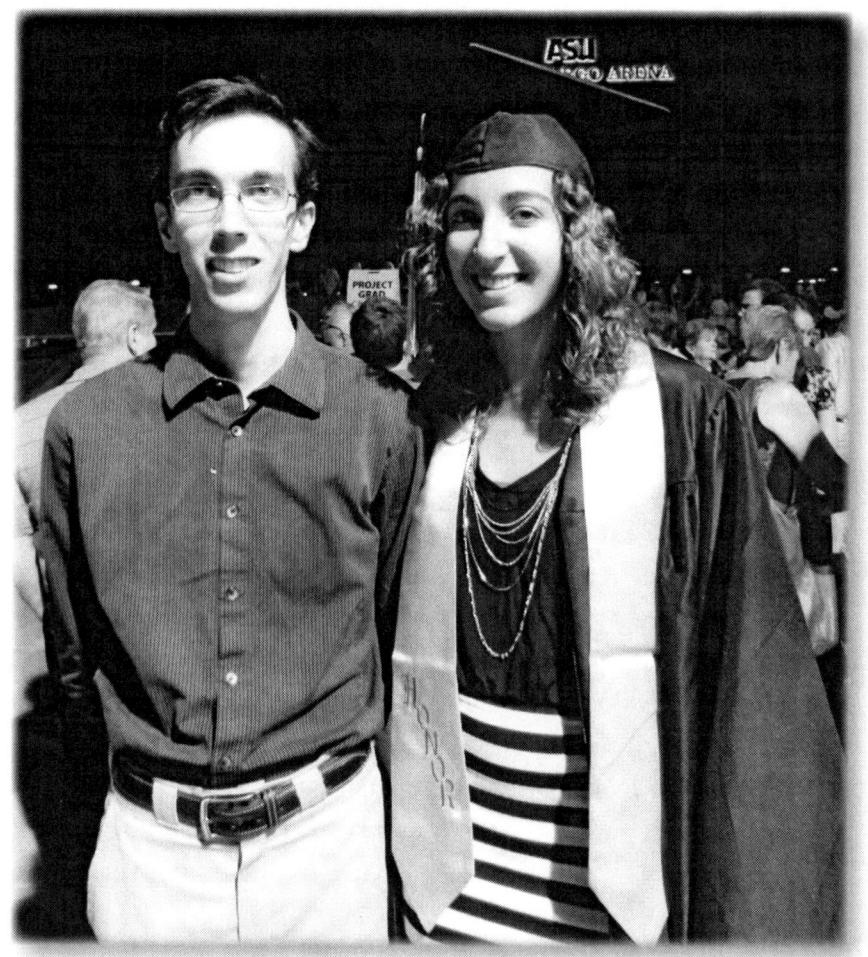

Brian and Emily, at her graduation.

we've been even more impressed by the character she's demonstrated during this most difficult school year of her young life.

One week after classes began last August, my breast cancer diagnosis detonated under our family like a roadside bomb. Emily was shocked and shaken, and though we reassured her that I would get the best treatment available, she knew there were no guarantees. As she ground through another year of honors classes, prepared her college applications, refereed soccer games, and socialized with friends, worry was her constant companion. My illness was an extra layer of stress on top of the usual pressures of senior year.

I felt really bad about how my cancer affected the family, but Emily was having none of that. She got angry at the disease, but never at me. She wrote me letters of encouragement, gave me hugs and 'girl time' every day, and participated in the Race for the Cure in my honor. Though she cried and vented her frustrations at times throughout the year, she always collected herself afterward and carried on. Maybe she knew that was the best thing she could do for me.

Emily arrived at graduation a stronger, wiser person than the girl who began senior year last summer. The adversities of the past nine months made her grow. One of the speakers at the commencement ceremony told a story about a wheelchair-bound man nearing the end of a self-propelled journey around the world. Along his path, a little girl held up a sign that said, "The end is the beginning."

I listened to that story and thought about how far my family has traveled since August. Now that my treatment is over and I am still here, getting healthier and more energetic every day, the worry lines have disappeared from their faces. The end is the beginning.

June Feels Good!

Monday, June 4, 2012

To look at me these days, you might never know I spent most of the past year fighting cancer. My hair is long enough to pass for a short hairstyle, my skin has regained its usual pinkish hue, and the joint stiffness that plagued me for months has disappeared. Fatigue, which settled over me like an afternoon cloud during radiation, has blown away.

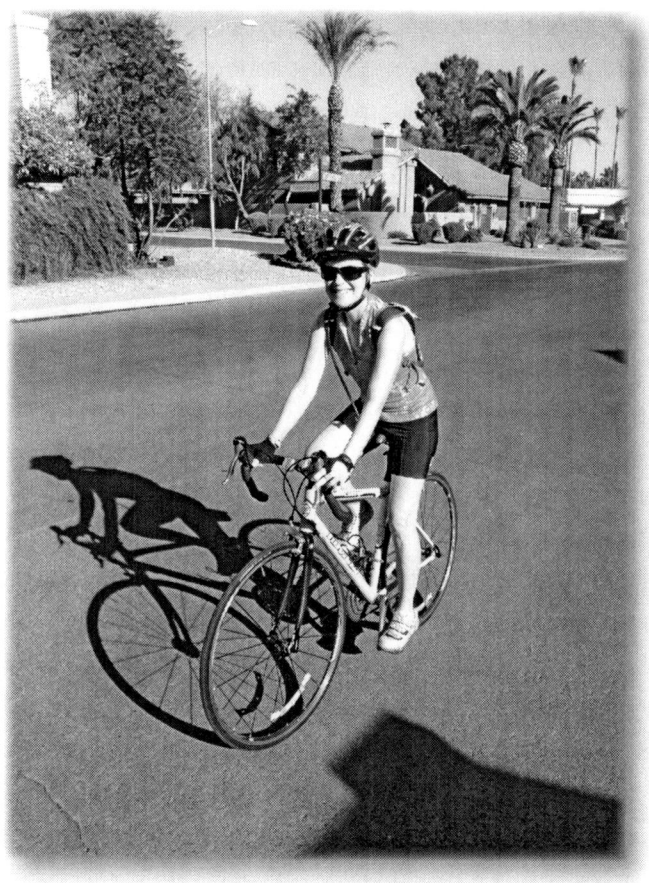

The best thing about a prolonged, serious illness is how great it feels to regain your health. A few weeks ago, after a nine-month hiatus due to cancer, I got back on my road bike. I've since been on some twenty-mile rides, without problems. My left arm shows no signs of lymphedema, the swelling that can occur following lymph node removal and radiation. Yoga, my newest activity, is helping rebuild strength and flexibility in that arm and the rest of my body. Gradually, my speed while hiking up the mountains is improving. I may never be as fast as before chemo and radiation, but I have hope.

Tamoxifen, the estrogen-blocking pill I've been taking daily for almost a month, seems to agree with me. I get hot flashes and dry skin, which are minor issues when compared with the trials of the past year. A hot flash is no sweat (or perhaps only a little more sweat) for a woman who hikes all summer in Phoenix.

While delighted to be feeling good and getting back to a normal life, I still can't go for more than a few hours without thinking about breast cancer. Maybe that is the "new normal" for me. In the next month or so, my doctors and I will be making some decisions about my ongoing care, such as what screening tests are appropriate for my remaining breast. One doctor recommends both mammogram and MRI once a year, six months apart, for the next two years.

Later this month, my other oncologist will weigh in on screening and other treatment options. I want to ask him more questions about the bone-strengthening drug Zometa (Reclast). Last time we met, he said preliminary studies showed a 30 percent reduction of recurrence in breast cancer patients like me who had intravenous infusions of Zometa. The women studied had infusions every six months for two years. I cringe at the thought of more infusions and the inevitable side effects of yet another drug. At the same time, who wouldn't want to reduce her chance of recurrence by 30 percent?

Between now and that doctor's appointment, Moe and I are traveling to Hawaii—our reward to ourselves for enduring cancer treatment. We'll be staying on Kauai, the "garden island," a place to forget about cancer if ever there was one. A week from today, we'll be paddling a kayak along the Na Pali Coast, a lush, steep landscape of coves, waterfalls, and rainbows. After surgery on my chest and armpit in February, I didn't imagine I'd be operating a paddle by June. We planned our trip expecting to hang out on the beach and watch sunsets. A few weeks ago, however, Moe and I rented a two-person kayak on a local lake and discovered we make a champion paddling team. Na Pali, here we come.

cf cf cf

Below is one of my blog posts from the island of Kauai, Hawaii, an ideal locale for recovering from the mental and physical rigors of cancer treatment.

Greetings from Paradise

Monday, June 11, 2012

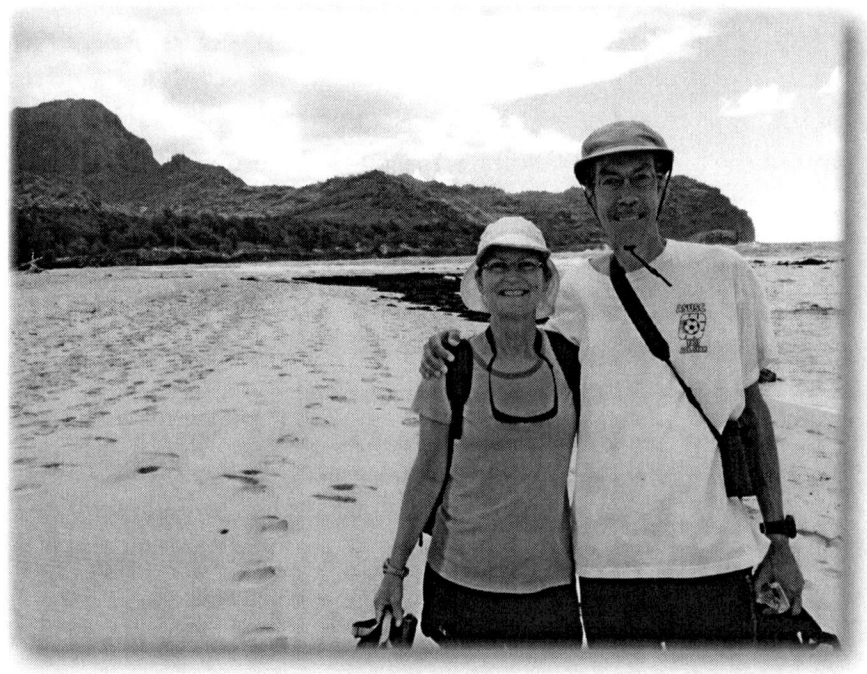

Kauai, Hawaii

Today, Moe and I paid $5 each to enter Kilauea Point Wildlife Refuge, and departed an hour later with a guarantee of "good luck for life." I call that a good value.

Kauai's Kilauea Point, a high bluff overlooking the Pacific Ocean, is the northernmost tip of the Hawaiian Islands. A historic lighthouse resides there, as well as the modern beacon light that replaced it in the 1970s. A fantastic selection of seabirds also live on the cliffs of Kilauea Point: white tropicbirds with tube-like ten-inch red or white tails, black great frigate birds with forked tails and menacing speed, red-footed boobies whose white bodies are accented by red feet and blue bills, gray wedge-tailed shearwaters that shyly nest in the bushes, and the Laysan albatross, a huge white flyer trimmed in black.

According to a refuge naturalist, a close-up view of an albatross brings good luck for life, and Kilauea Point is one of only a few places on land where you can see one. She suggested we point our binoculars toward the bird's dirt "landing strip" on the adjoining cliff, and wait for mama albatross to fly in after a long day filling up at the ocean's all-you-can-eat buffet.

Not five minutes later, the bird glided overhead, circled the point a few times, and skidded to a stop in the dirt. This creature has a wingspan of seventy-eight inches, and while graceful in flight, barely flapping its wings, it appears awkward on land. Hence the nickname "Gooney Bird." The Laysan albatross was one of five "life birds" Moe spotted today. He was one happy birdman. I was much more focused on the unexpected and much appreciated good luck component of today's adventure.

Albatrosses have survived on earth for twenty-five million years. Some of them lay eggs and raise young for more than sixty years. Seems to me this species has good fortune to spare, and I hope some rubs off on this new graduate of cancer treatment.

Postscript: My friend Judy commented, "Red-footed boobies? Really? Is there a more appropriate bird sighting for a breast cancer survivor? I suppose the picture in my head, of breasts waddling around on red duck feet, is probably not accurate, but I hope you got a good laugh out of it just the same."

Judy's image of breasts on duck feet cracked me up, but until she pointed it out, I had completely missed the joke. I went to Hawaii to get away from thoughts of breasts, boobies, mammary glands, or whatever you want to call them. For me, the red-footed boobies were only birds.

A Brief Encounter with "The Monster"

Saturday, June 30, 2012

A few months ago, while I was still having radiation treatments, my medical oncologist mentioned the bone-strengthening drug Zometa (Reclast). In preliminary studies, he explained, Zometa has reduced recurrence of breast cancer by as much as 30 percent in patients like me.

"Look it up on the Internet and we'll talk about it next time," he said.

Moe and I read up on Zometa, and the reviews were mixed. Some studies found less breast cancer recurrence in women who used the drug, while other studies showed little or no effect. The course of treatment proposed for me would involve an intravenous infusion of Zometa every six months for two years. Each infusion would likely cause short-term bone pain, though the drug is tolerated well by most people. Rare complications like jaw necrosis (bone death) can affect people with dental problems, so you need a clean bill of health from your dentist before starting the infusions.

The two of us went to Dr. K.'s office on June 21, uncertain about Zometa. I asked the doctor straight out whether he would recommend this drug for me, even though it's not fully proven. Without hesitation he said, "I would absolutely recommend it for you. Your cancer was ugly, still in a few lymph nodes even after chemo. Anything that might help prevent recurrence is a good idea."

The doctor's message was painful to hear. I know my cancer was bad, but have spent months trying to be positive and not let fear get the best of me. "Your cancer was ugly" rang in my ears and made my stomach clench. "The Monster," an evil presence that tries to suck the hope from anyone battling a life-threatening illness, entered the exam room on the back of those four words.

My doctor had no idea, and I didn't tell him. Instead, I asked how soon I should start the Zometa. He said the sooner, the better. Moe and I scheduled my first infusion for July 18.

In the car on the way home, I let out some tears and lamented to my husband about receiving mixed messages. This same doctor has estimated my chances of recurrence at 15 to 20 percent, but when I went to his office and heard "Your cancer was ugly," it felt as though recurrence was a foregone conclusion. I have to remind myself that it's not. When I'm afraid, I have to thrust my indomitable spirit into The Monster's face like a mortal holds up a cross to fend off a vampire.

At each visit, my doctor checks for signs of cancer during the physical exam. Every six months, he orders a blood test that looks for cancer in my bloodstream. There will be regular mammograms and/or MRIs in my future, too. I am learning to manage the anxiety that accompanies such tests. Dr. K. sees worst-case scenarios every day, but that doesn't mean I will be one. I am going for "best-case scenario" status.

On the prevention side of things, the oncologist has recommended every strategy he knows to thwart recurrence—Tamoxifen, Zometa, and the healthiest lifestyle I can manage. I am doing everything I can to stay well, receiving excellent medical care, and feeling great. Take that, Monster, and crawl back into your hole!

Postscript: My friend Laura, a fellow breast cancer survivor, wrote, "Carrie, thank you for sharing this experience. We can all get a bit down when someone we trust uses hard words. Looking up and not down is the right Rx."

She's right. What you tell yourself about your condition, and the words you use in describing it to others, affects your quality of life. During treatment and since, I have strived to cast my situation in the best possible light, and to stamp out negative thoughts with positive ones. It's not always easy, but mostly it works.

My husband tells a cautionary tale of a woman whose breast cancer was already in the lymph nodes before it was discovered, much like mine. Though her doctors questioned whether she would survive, the patient responded well to treatment. After surgery, chemo, and radiation, she was cancer free, but also depressed. She didn't like her body after treatment. She assumed her cancer would recur, and she worried about it continually. "Why me?" she complained to anyone and everyone. The woman is now a two-decade survivor, but her depression persists to this day.

If only she had learned to look up and not down.

Visiting My "VIPs"

Sunday, July 8, 2012

Last fall, I wrote that a cancer diagnosis brings clarity about what's most important in life. At the top of my most-important list were "people, relationships, and experiences."

During months of treatment, I often thought of the people I most wanted to visit when the ordeal was over. Not surprisingly,

Mom and Dad were the first people who came to mind. My second post-treatment trip, after the Hawaiian getaway with Moe, would be to Reno, Nevada (Dad's home) and Wenatchee, Washington (Mom's summer residence).

I am on that journey now, accompanied by my eighteen-year-old daughter, Emily. We landed in Wenatchee yesterday, after a few days in Reno that my father described as "the best visit we've ever had." It's true. An in-person heart-to-heart with Dad was precious to me, especially after two years apart and a bout with cancer. I know he felt the same. We have always been close, but appreciated our time together more than ever.

I was glad to arrive in Reno with my health restored and a full head of hair, and not just for Dad. His younger daughter, eighteen-year-old Dani, lost her mother to breast cancer five years ago. Last fall, she was afraid she might lose her big sister, too. I wanted to show her what a survivor looks like. She and my father are counting on me to stay well, and I don't intend to disappoint.

Deja Vu

Wednesday, July 18, 2012

Today I had an uncomfortable sense of deja vu as I found myself back in the chemotherapy suite at my oncologist's office. I was there for a twenty-minute infusion of Zometa, the bone-strengthening drug that may reduce my chances of cancer recurrence by as much as 30 percent. As the nurse slid the IV needle into a vein in my left arm, I glanced around at the dozen or more occupied recliners lining the room. Men and women with thinning hair, bald, or sporting hats or wigs sat patiently, taking their medicines, fighting their cancers. Seven months ago, I was just like them, hoping for a cure via the hanging bags of chemo drugs fed into my body by a tube and a port in my chest.

This afternoon, I was probably the healthiest-looking patient in the room. Oh how I hope to stay that way. Nurse Angie seemed to understand what was going through my mind.

"I wonder when I'll stop thinking about cancer all the time and worrying about recurrence," I said.

"Never," she said. Though she hasn't had cancer, this experienced chemo nurse admitted that she's always checking herself for signs of it. Cancer paranoia is perhaps an inevitable byproduct of her job.

As she left to tend to other patients, I pulled my reading material out of my bag, and felt even more determined to live life fully and without regret. I thought back to last week, when I rode a passenger ferry with my mother and daughter into the wilderness at the north end of fifty-five-mile-long Lake Chelan in Washington. In the tiny village of Stehekin, a place with no roads connecting to the outside world, we rode a shuttle bus a few miles to soaring Rainbow Falls. After a record snow year in the Cascades and a recent heat wave, water careened over the cliff with an awesome fury. We loved the miles of clear blue lake, timbered slopes, and glacier-topped peaks in the distance, but the falls were the highlight we will all remember. That, and the time together—mother, daughter, and granddaughter. Just the thought of it brought a smile to my lips.

Postscript: My pal Karen commented, "When does the friend of a cancer survivor stop thinking about her friend and her experiences with, and worries about, the disease? Never! Still reading, and with you long-distance in thought and prayer. Thanks for sharing your intention to live joyfully and with zest, appreciating each person, experience, and insight."

When you're a cancer patient (or a recent survivor), it's easy to become wrapped up in your own thoughts and feelings. Battling a life-threatening illness is an intense experience that sometimes takes every bit of energy you have. And yet, as Karen's words reminded me, the experience is NOT all about you. How you're doing and the outcome of your treatment impacts everyone who knows and cares about you.

This perspective is important. My loved ones deserve more from me than self-absorption and a continual monologue of my worries about cancer. They need to see me move forward in my life and be available to cheer them on through their life challenges. That's when they'll know my recovery is complete.

In the last six months of 2012, my blog posts became fewer and farther between as I began taking baby steps toward what I hoped would be a cancer-free future. With the crisis of treatment past, it was time to start looking outside of myself.

Too Much Is Better than Too Little

Thursday, August 2, 2012

Two weeks ago today, I headed off on a morning bike ride with my girlfriends. My first Zometa infusion had been the day before, and I was hoping to be one of those lucky people with no side effects. Though feeling a little "off" at breakfast, I was sure a twenty-mile ride would put me right.

It didn't. I struggled the whole way. At the top of the hill, as I stood over my bike gulping water and trying to make conversation with Pam and Melissa, my eyes drifted to a shady patch of hot pavement. *If only I could curl up there and rest a while.*

Recognizing my distress, Melissa suggested we ride the short distance to her house so she could drive me home. A few hours later, I was lying on my living room couch, wrapped in a hoodie and blanket despite 109-degree heat outside. The fever and chills passed in a few hours, followed by fatigue and mild bone pain.

I made a note to self: *Do not plan strenuous activity the day after a Zometa infusion.* I'll try to remember that in six months, when it's time for the next one.

Fortunately, my body bounces back quickly. By Friday, I was well enough (sort of) to go camping with Moe. While hardly eager to sleep on the ground in a tiny tent after a day of fever and aches, I made myself go. Moe had a campsite reserved at the Rose Canyon Lake campground on the slopes of Mount Lemmon, a hangout of the reclusive buff-breasted flycatcher.

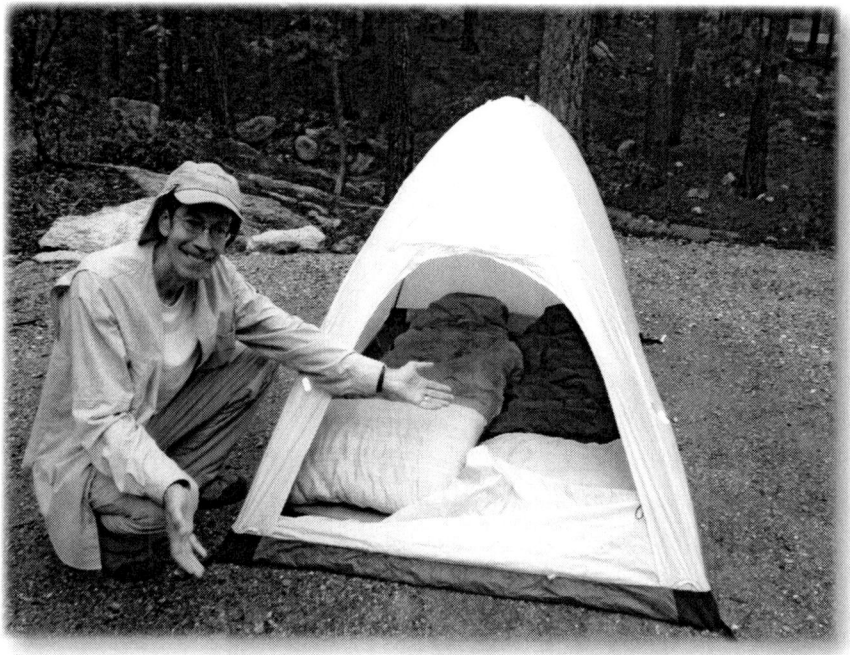

I had forgotten how much I enjoy camping. How magical it can be to step outside the tent at midnight and look up at a starry sky, awake to the dawn chorus of birdsong, and see a dramatic natural landscape for the first time. Catalina Highway, the winding road that climbs from the desert floor of Tucson to the alpine slopes of Mount Lemmon, features jagged cliffs, hoodoos, and panoramic vistas.

We spotted nearly twenty different bird species around Rose Canyon, but never got a good look at our target bird. "That's okay," I told my disappointed birdman, "because it means we get to go back."

During chemo last year, I made myself get up and out of the house even when I didn't feel good. It was so much better to be outside on a trail than confined to the easy chair in front of the TV. Even now, if I err on the side of doing too much after a trying medical event, I think that's better than doing too little. The bike ride may have been pushing it, but I'm glad I went camping.

Full Circle

Tuesday, August 14, 2012

A few days ago, I attended an annual writing conference organized by a mystery writers' group of which I am a member. I was hoping the speakers would fire me up to re-engage in my half-finished mystery novel. I entered the hotel ballroom with aspirations, but also with trepidation.

Last year, I went to this same event shortly after learning I had cancer. I remember well the bittersweet feelings that passed through me during and after that day. The keynote speakers were three successful female crime novelists. Exuding wit and humor, they pumped up the audience with inspiration and how-to. The overall message was, "If we could do it, you can do it, and here's how." I sat in that room with friends from my writer's critique group, hanging on the speakers' every word, buying into the message. Just as I began to believe it, the reality of my situation dawned. *You have cancer. You start chemo next week.*

What a difference a year makes. I barely looked at my novel. It didn't seem important while I was fighting cancer. For me, the past year was about enduring treatment, facing down the fear of death, growing as a person during a difficult passage in life, and appreciating the amazing generosity and love of friends and family.

While I have been changed by my year with cancer, I don't want to be defined by it. A few weeks ago, I celebrated my first birthday post-cancer. It felt like a signal to get back to my normal life, a cancer-free existence in which I might write fiction, travel to distant lands, and help others on their cancer journeys.

With all this in mind, I went to the conference, got reacquainted with writing friends I hadn't seen in a year, and found the encouragement I was looking for. One of the keynote speakers was a successful film and TV writer before becoming a psychologist specializing in creative people. Most of the patients on his couch are writers plagued by problems such as self-doubt, writer's block, deadline anxiety, envy of more successful writers, and procrastination. This writers' shrink, who is also a mystery author, has seen it all and has cultivated the art of turning negative thoughts into positive ones.

The following are a few of his pearls of wisdom: 1) For those of us who think we are lacking something, "You are enough to be the **writer** (or fill in the blank) you want to be." 2) "The writer's enemy is the search for inspiration. It's already inside you. Rather than waiting for inspiration, cultivate imagination." 3) "Writing begets writing. Do not allow yourself not to write!"

Great advice. It made me want to finish the book I started and believe that it is possible.

A Good Hair Day

Wednesday, August 15, 2012

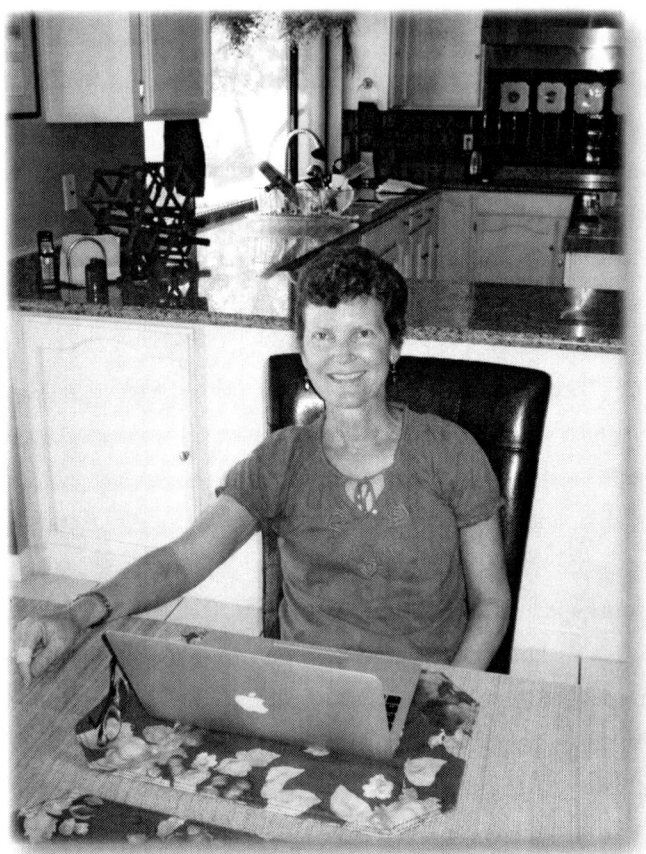

Yesterday I had my first haircut in eleven months. Our hairdresser, Iva, who shaved off my chemo-scorched locks last September and refused payment, made quick work of cleaning up the lush curls that now carpet my head. If last year's buzz cut got me ready to do battle with cancer, yesterday's trim was all about sprucing up to enjoy renewed health. The timing couldn't have been better.

Today is the one-year anniversary of my cancer diagnosis, a day that shall live in infamy in my world. You'd think it might be a sad day, evoking unpleasant memories, but that is not the case. I feel reborn today. Maybe it's because I have emerged from a dark and difficult year, and back into the light. Perhaps it's because the cancer monkey is off my back. Or it could just be the haircut.

A New Life Passage

Wednesday, August 29, 2012

The past two weeks have brought big changes to the Bell house. After a year-and-a-half break, our son Brian has gone back to college. Believe me, this is cause for celebration. Brian needed time, space and encouragement while he figured things out. Those items were not always easy to give. Sometimes our house felt too small to hold a moody young adult and his frustrated parents. My cancer episode didn't help matters. I'm glad now that we waited him out.

Brian is attending school locally and still living at home, something Moe and I don't mind, especially now that his sister has gone to California to begin her own college career. That is the other big change around here. We traveled to Los Angeles over the weekend to attend freshman orientation with Emily at our alma mater, Occidental College. Moe and I were happy, sad, and nostalgic as we moved our daughter into her cubicle in Braun Hall, located next door to the dormitory where both of us spent our freshman years.

In our mind's eye, we see her treading the familiar path up the hill between the quad and her dorm. We picture her in all of our old haunts—the student union, library, quadrangle, classrooms, and athletic fields. We take comfort in knowing her surroundings; we believe she is at a school that is the right "fit." And yet, as Moe said following our return to Arizona without Emily on Sunday, "There is a little hole in my heart." Mine too. Our girl has entered a new passage in her life, one in which her parents will play a much reduced role.

At the same time, we begin our own next phase of life, one that (we hope) will involve fewer responsibilities at home and more time for travel. Having Brian here makes the transition a little easier, as he can hold down the fort while we're away. Our first stop is Ireland. We leave tomorrow night.

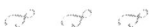

Below is one of several posts from our ten days in Ireland:

It's a Long Way from Chemo to the Cliffs of Moher

Sunday, September 2, 2012

It's late and we're tired, but I couldn't let this night go by without a short comment. A year ago today, I started chemotherapy for breast cancer. The future seemed very uncertain.

Today, I hiked ten miles with my husband from the tiny village of Doolin, Ireland to the Cliffs of Moher and back. Walking along the cliff tops with the wind in my face and the sound of the Atlantic surf rolling up against the rocks below, I remembered where I was last year at this time. Now is so much better than then, and I am so grateful.

Tonight, Moe and I are in Galway, just back from "Trad on the Prom," a show featuring traditional Irish music and dance. Think Riverdance meets The Chieftains, only live and not on a PBS pledge drive weekend. In fact, a lot of the performers actually *were* from Riverdance, The Chieftains, and Lord of the Dance. I have fallen in love with the Irish uilleann pipes. That is the instrument you hear in the theme song for *Titanic*. We'll go to sleep with the pipes' soulful wail still in our ears.

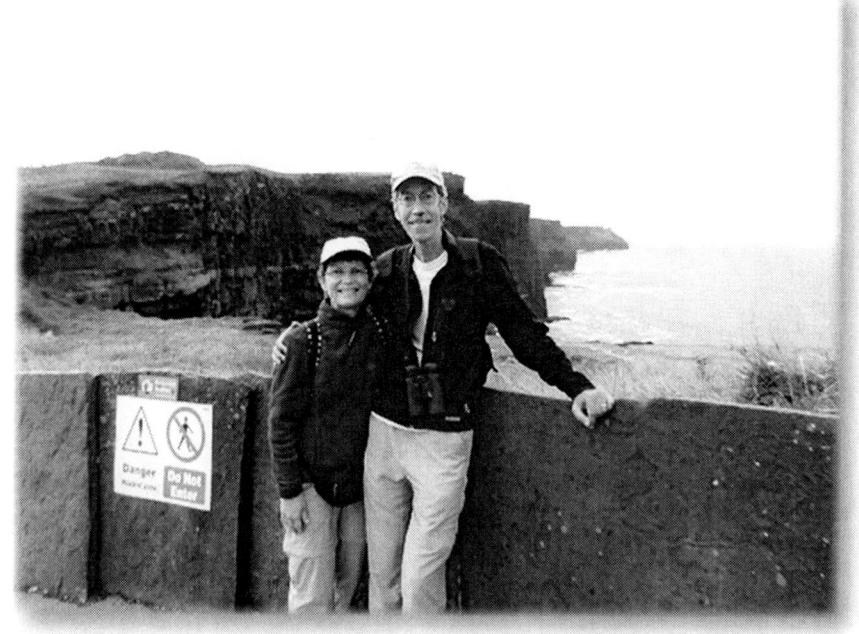

At Cliffs of Moher, western Ireland.

Dreams Can Come True

Friday, October 5, 2012

Last October, while undergoing chemotherapy, I missed out on my annual trek across the Grand Canyon. *Next year, I'll be back*, I thought. I pictured being on the trail, watching the sunrise light up the soaring rock walls. It was a pleasant dream that helped me through a bleak time.

Finally, "next year" has arrived. In a few hours, my friends and I will be driving north toward Arizona's high country and that big hole in the ground that takes everyone's breath away. Since returning from Ireland, I've spent many hours on the trail preparing to hike from rim to rim once more.

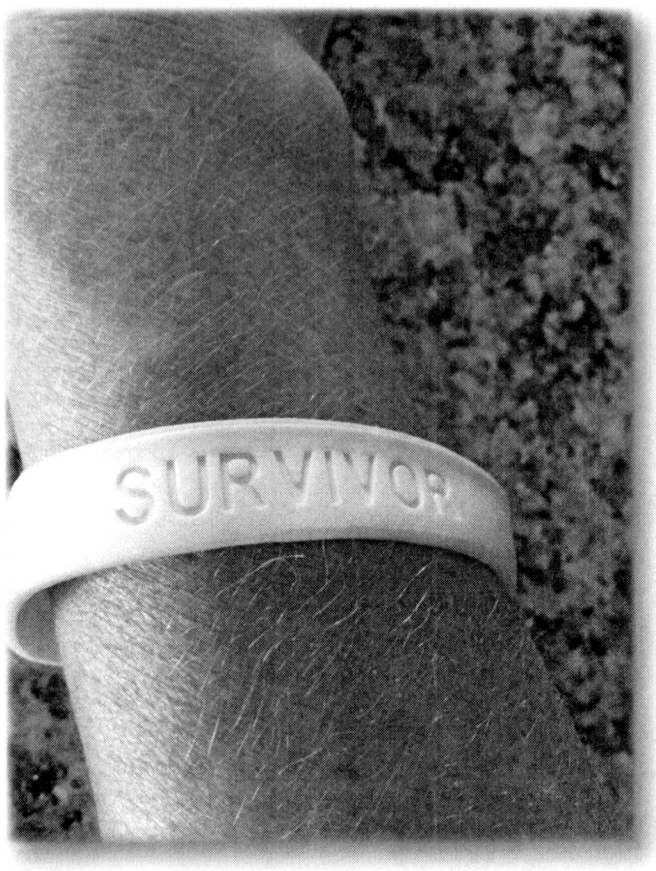

I'll be wearing the "survivor" bracelet I received yesterday after getting my first mammogram since before cancer treatment. "You are A-OK," the technician said after the mammogram and a thorough ultrasound of my "very dense and fibrous" remaining breast. I slipped on my new bracelet while swallowing the lump in my throat. On Saturday, when I am walking the twenty-one miles from the South Rim to the North Rim, I will look at that little pink band on my arm and be reminded of just how far I've come since last October.

Postscript: Friends cheered me on after reading this post. Karen wrote, "You are awesome! I will be thinking of you and this marvelous journey every step of the way." Gayle said, "This post brings tears to my eyes. What a journey it has been for you."

Yep, it's been absolutely life changing.

Victory March

Wednesday, October 10, 2012

"A journey of a thousand miles begins with a single step."

–Lao Tzu

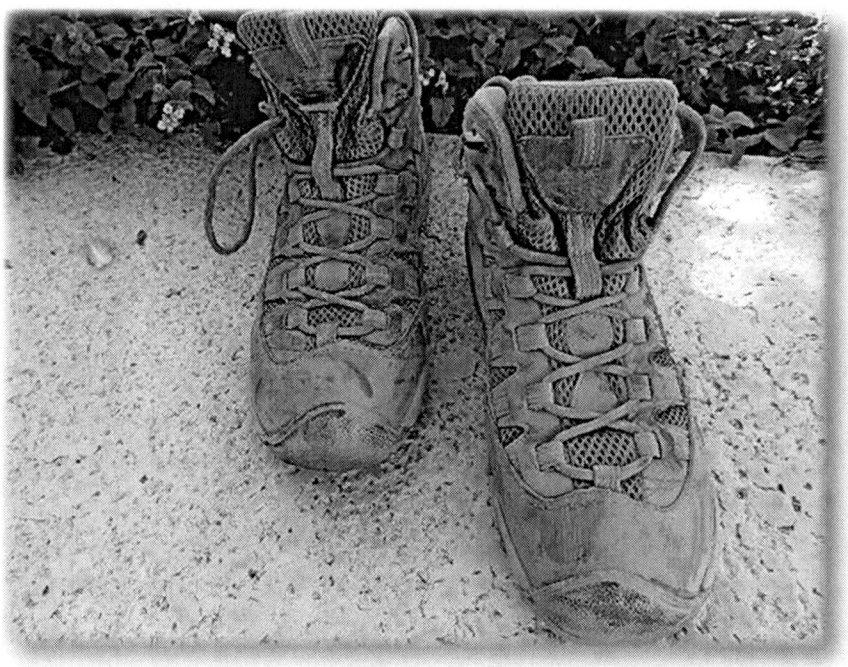

My "new" boots, baptized in Grand Canyon trail dust.

This past weekend, my journey of forty-two miles back and forth across the Grand Canyon began and ended with a single step—not to mention many thousands in between.

Saturday, South Rim to North Rim: We started our twenty-one-mile trek on the South Kaibab Trail at 4:40 a.m. Pam and Angie, my workout partners throughout the year, were by my side once again. These BFFs did this hike with me in 2009 and 2010. Last time, high winds and rain turned the last leg of our adventure into a miserable ordeal. We emerged from the canyon sodden from head to toe.

"Never again," Pam said afterward.

"I had to get cancer to get you to come back," I teased a few months ago, when she agreed to do the trip a third time.

Another good friend, Melissa, volunteered to be our driver this year. When she dropped us off at the trailhead in the dark, we were greeted by a familiar stiff breeze. Our headlamps illuminated dust particles swirling in the air, a rocky powder ground fine by mule trains that travel the path daily. Twenty yards down the trail I could already feel grit crunching against my teeth. *Ah, so good to be back!* I thought.

South Kaibab Trail, with its serpentine switchbacks, is steep, rugged, and unrelenting for seven miles. Between the South Rim and Phantom Ranch, the tiny enclave of civilization at the bottom of the canyon, the trail drops 4,760 feet. Hiking poles, planted with each step, kept our middle-aged knees from breaking down during the wicked descent.

On the plus side, the trail provided incomparable views. There is no prettier sight than sunrise over the Grand Canyon from South Kaibab Trail. A few times, I have seen the full moon setting to my left while the sun rose over the canyon to my right. Sublime is the only word for it, despite the accompanying sweat and grit.

Recovery

I usually push the pace coming down SK Trail, but not this year. Cancer has taught me to savor each moment. My friends were a bit shocked to find me stopping to take pictures and not checking my watch during each bathroom break.

Our threesome strolled into Phantom Ranch after three-and-a-half hours—a slow time by my usual standards, but so what? We arrived just as the cafe opened, and were able to purchase three tall glasses of freshly brewed iced tea. Seven miles down, fourteen to go.

Revitalized by trail food, caffeinated sport beans, and iced tea, the Three Amigas bolted out of Phantom Ranch on the North Kaibab Trail toward Cottonwood Campground as if our day had just begun. In no time, we were in "the box," crossing back and forth over Bright Angel Creek in a narrow canyon bordered by steep rock walls. Somewhere in the middle, fatigue began to set in.

"Are there five bridges across the creek, or six?"

"How much farther to Cottonwood, do you think?"

Unsatisfied with my answers, Pam and Angie distracted themselves by singing the theme songs of TV shows from the '60s and '70s. *The Brady Bunch*, *The Beverly Hillbillies*, *Gilligan's Island* ... Angie knows them all. (OK, I know them, too.) Pam spent hours trying to master the lyrics to *The Brady Bunch*, much to the amusement and consternation of passing hikers.

"What were they singing?" I heard one young man ask his companions. I had dropped behind the gals to adjust my pack. "It's *The Brady Bunch*," I said unapologetically. "It passes the time."

Three hours of mildly uphill walking brought us to Cottonwood Campground, where I refilled my empty 100-ounce Camelback bladder and wolfed a lunch of sunflower bagel and cream cheese. Fourteen miles down, seven to go—the last and hardest part of our canyon crossing with a 4,200-foot climb.

In my mind, I break this last leg into smaller sections: Two miles from Cottonwood to the artist's house (a ranger outpost with bathroom and water); two miles from the artist's house to Three-mile Bridge; one mile from Three-mile Bridge to Supai Tunnel; two miles from Supai Tunnel to the North Rim. Between Cottonwood and the North Rim, I've seen hikers succumb to heat exhaustion, blisters, and sore muscles. I hoped I was up to the challenge.

At the artist's house (an artist and his family lived there for two decades), I was worried. Two uphill miles in full sun on a full stomach had not agreed with me. While my pals used the facilities, I popped sport beans, sucked thirstily from my water tube, and hoped for the best. A cooling breeze, increasing shade, and dropping temperatures as we neared the alpine climes of the North Rim saved the day for me.

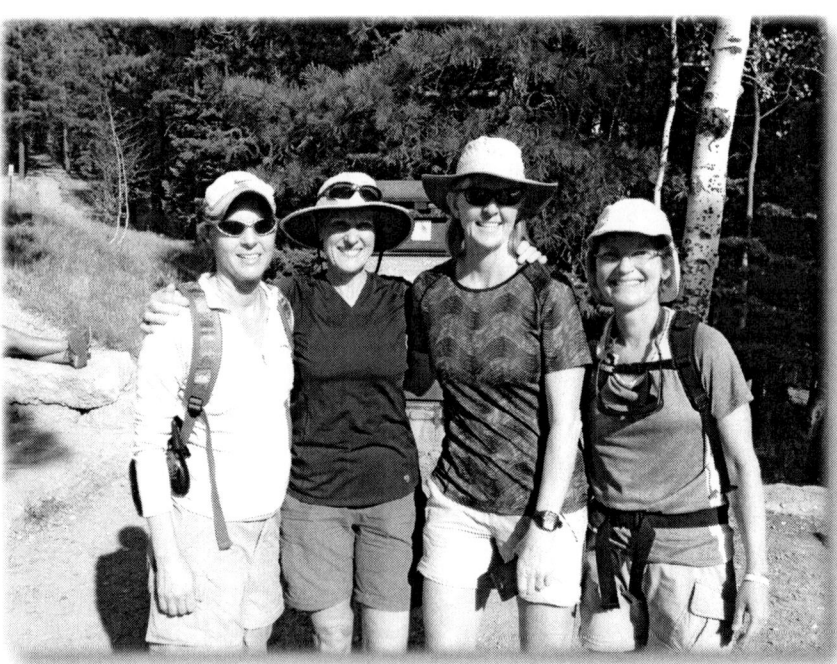

Left to right: Melissa, Pam, Angie, and me at North Rim trailhead.

Recovery

Since cancer, chemo, surgery, and radiation, I struggle a bit on super-steep terrain under a hot sun. On Saturday, I got the super-steep, but not the super-hot. My team reached the North Rim in high spirits ten and a half hours after departing the South Rim. It's hard to describe the joy of that moment. Less than six months after radiation, it felt like a victory—over cancer, fears that I might never be the same, and the physical and psychological hurdles that must be overcome following a life-threatening illness. There was no doubt in my mind that I would be able to make the return trip to the South Rim on Monday.

After a day of rest, including an hour-long stretch massage that gave new life to my feet and legs, and hangout time with canyon friends made during many years of October rim-to-rim-to-rim treks, we arose Monday in the wee hours of the morning and retraced our

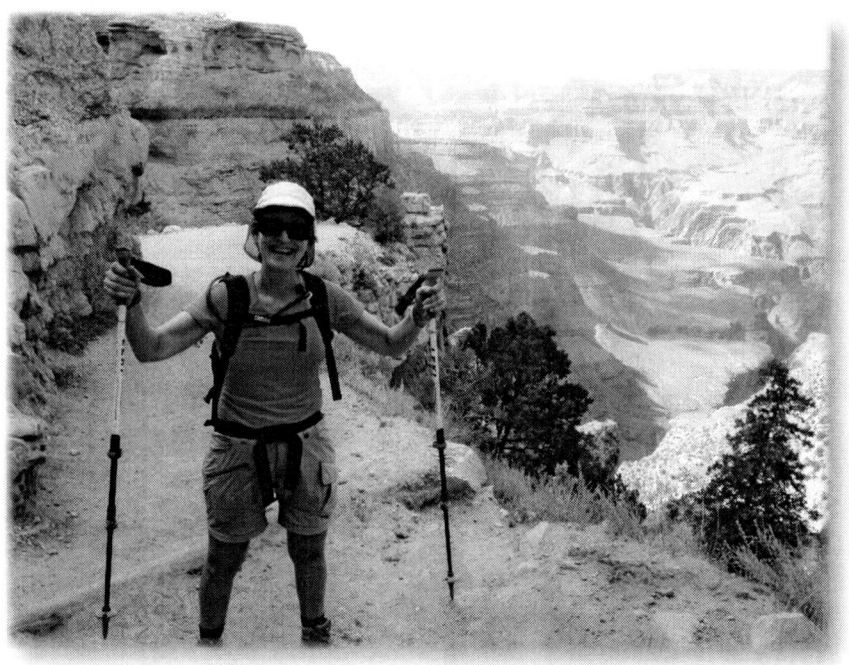

Victory! My fourteenth rim-to-rim-to-rim is complete.

steps. Our group emerged triumphant on the South Rim ten hours later.

At my lowest moment on Monday, after trudging up the steepest, hottest section of SK Trail, when it all seemed too damned hard, my companions heaped encouragement upon me, punctuated by a loud eruption of trail flatulence (I won't say from whom). I nearly fell down laughing, and all tension and frustration vanished from my being. Somehow these friends always know what I need, and manage to provide it. I hope I do the same for them. Thank you Pam, Angie, and Melissa for sharing this year's canyon experience with me. I will treasure the memories forever.

Postscript: Cancer not only makes you fear for your life, it also makes you worry about what you might lose permanently due to treatment. Like other women ravaged from fighting breast cancer, I wondered whether I would ever again feel feminine or attractive. A loving husband helped me overcome that concern. Another big unknown was whether my body would be healthy enough to allow continuation of the active outdoor lifestyle that I love. Completing the rim-to-rim-to-rim trek in the Grand Canyon less than a year after chemo answered the latter question with a resounding, "Yes."

Reflections on Gratitude from a Breast Cancer Survivor

Sunday, October 14, 2012

I am grateful for…

1. Strength, health, and being cancer-free.
2. The opportunity to participate in the Race for the Cure as a "one-year survivor."

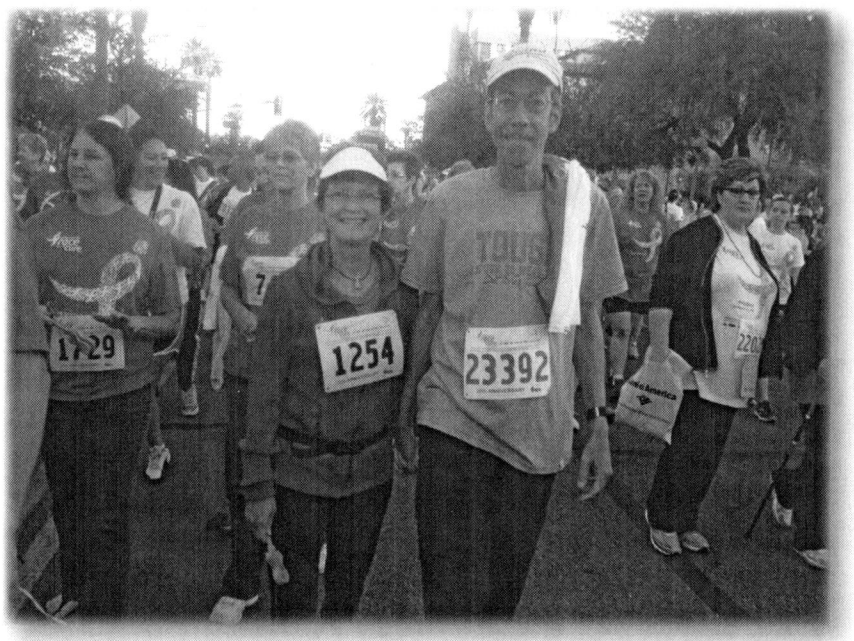

With Moe at Race for the Cure—Phoenix, this morning.

3. The love of family and friends. Who would want to be a survivor without that?

4. The doctors, nurses, techs, treatments, and research that helped me overcome a very serious episode of breast cancer.

5. The world's best husband, my "co-survivor," who has been by my side in the valleys and the shadows, as well as the sunshine.

6. The privilege to hike once again in the Grand Canyon last weekend, watching the golden sunrise over the South Rim on Saturday and observing the stars, countless brilliant greetings from light-years away, twinkling over the North Rim early Monday morning. As I walked through the canyon's ancient rock layers, I was reminded once again of my humble position in this world.

7. The lessons of cancer. Since last year's illness, I am more present in each moment, worry less about things I cannot control, and have learned to conquer my fears. I have let go of past regrets, stopped sweating the small stuff, and place a much higher value on experiences than possessions. I have received love in abundance and have plenty to give.

Though I wouldn't wish this disease on anyone, for me, personal growth has been the silver lining—another type of awareness to focus upon during Breast Cancer Awareness Month.

Postscript: Moe and I participated in Race for the Cure again the following October. As a "two-year survivor," I expected to be less moved and less emotional during the event than I had been the previous year. Who was I kidding? Upon taking my place in the Survivors Parade, my throat thickened and my eyes filled with tears. I couldn't speak for a while and surreptitiously wiped away the wet tracks on my cheeks. This happened a few more times, during breakfast at the Survivors Café and as we fast-walked the streets of Phoenix with the pink army.

Stop It! You've recovered from cancer. You don't cry about it anymore. Despite the shouting of my internal voice, I couldn't check the emotions sweeping over me. While I am grateful for my wonderful life as a survivor, sometimes I DO still cry over cancer. Maybe when there's a cure I'll be able to stop.

Survivors' Kinship

Tuesday, October 23, 2012

Ten days ago, I shared a table with a half-dozen other breast cancer warriors in the Survivors Café at the Race for the Cure. Some of us had been through chemo and radiation, some not. Some of us had

had lumpectomies to remove our tumors, and others mastectomies. Several of the survivors I met at the Komen Race had battled breast cancer more than once, a sobering realization for a newbie still traumatized by the first go-round.

Every breast cancer survivor has her own story. The lady on my right was a six-year survivor who'd had a mastectomy and chemo, and endured seven reconstructive surgeries before the doctors deemed her rebuilt boob and her real breast an acceptable match. Apparently, this is not uncommon. The next phase of my reconstruction is scheduled for December. I hope my plastic surgeon lives up to his excellent reputation.

The woman to my left had recently recovered from her second bout with breast cancer. "After the first time, I went skydiving with my daughter," she said. "It was something I had always wanted to do, and I loved it. The only thing I worried about was my daughter." After her second cancer battle, she started horseback riding several times a week. "Every day is precious," she said. "You should do the things you love to do." Everyone at our table nodded in agreement.

Even now, a week-and-a-half after the Race, I can still picture the faces of two other women I encountered at a booth offering free photographs for survivors. "Look," my husband said quietly, tilting his head toward a lady in front of us. She wore a pink ball cap over a fragile scalp just starting to sprout hair. The sight brought tears to my eyes. Only last spring, post-chemo, I looked like her.

Another face in the crowd belonged to a wife, mother, and two-time survivor who had driven to Phoenix from her home in Casa Grande, starting at 5 a.m., to be at the event in time for the Survivors Parade. She came because the Race for the Cure is her race; her life might depend on the next breakthrough.

I suspect that, like me, she felt a kinship with the other survivors, and drew strength and hope from the sight of thousands in pink filling the streets, walking and running in solidarity with us to defeat breast cancer. A few weeks ago, at the Grand Canyon, another two-time survivor told me, "You conquer cancer; cancer doesn't conquer you." Amen, sister.

Angel's Landing

Saturday, November 17, 2012

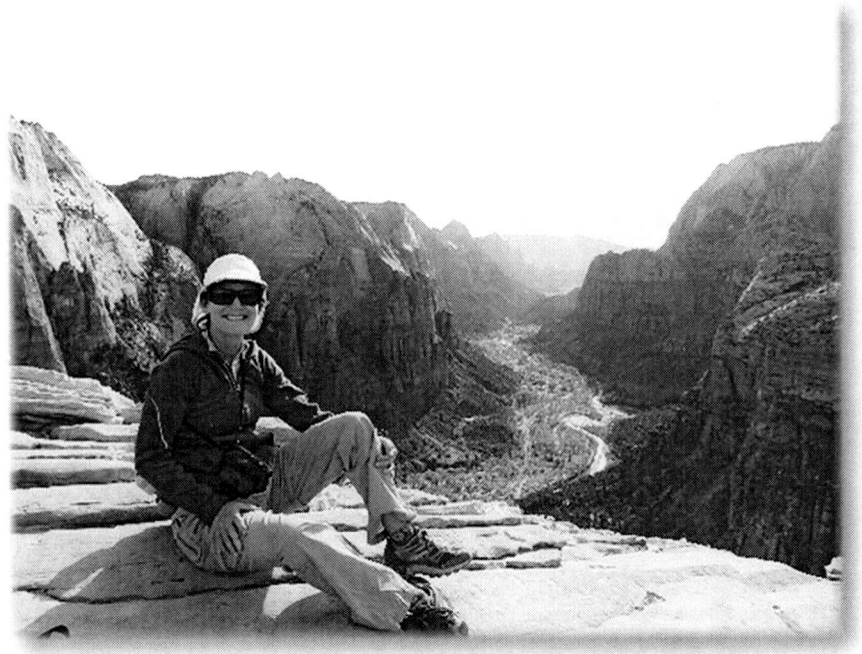

Atop Angel's Landing, Zion National Park.

Moe and I are in Utah's Zion National Park this week. I am trying to get my groove back with my mystery novel while he is attending a wilderness medicine conference. During his free time, we explore this canyon of towering red and buff slabs. It's been a great way to spend five days.

Thursday may have been our most memorable day here. Always on the lookout for a heart-thumping hike with stunning views at the top, we set out on an afternoon walk up 2.7-mile Angel's Landing Trail. Park literature describes this hike as strenuous and inappropriate for anyone with a fear of heights. Don't tell my mother, but a sign at the trailhead warns that six people have fallen to their death on this trail since 2004.

Chains are strung between metal poles sunk into the rock along the upper half-mile of the trail. The linked strands provide handholds across the narrow, uneven sandstone ridge you must traverse to reach the "landing." With 1,500-foot drops on either side of you, there is little room for error.

We agreed to start the hike and decide whether to continue once we got to the chains. Unlike most national park trails, this one was paved for the first two miles. While puffing up the side of a cliff along serpentine concrete switchbacks, Moe and I speculated on how the Park Service hauled cement up there.

As we ascended, sun-kissed vistas of majestic Zion Valley made us forget the pavement underfoot and our pounding hearts. In less than an hour, we emerged from the last set of switchbacks, Walter's Wriggles, and arrived at Scout's Landing. This is where you turn around if you have a fear of heights, aversion to risk, or a cautious personality.

My husband, while a cautious fellow in other respects, has a no-fear personality when it comes to climbing. Without a doubt, he would be continuing to Angel's Landing. I was not so sure. I have a mild fear of heights and am not brave in situations where a missed step is certain to result in death. In the past, I've turned back on dangerous slopes without ropes or chains to provide a measure of safety.

I studied the first chained section of trail beyond Scout's Landing and decided to keep going. Having something to hang on to gave me courage, though I will admit to a sick feeling in my stomach. A little while later, when I saw the long ridge that rose steeply from the saddle to the summit, my courage fled. "I'm not doing that," I said firmly.

A young woman behind us heard me. "You have to keep going," she said. "Nothing up there is harder than what you've already done."

She had been to Angel's Landing before, and spoke with authority. I surveyed the dicey ridge once more. Maybe it wasn't as bad as it looked. We pressed on. In several spots, the sandstone trail slopes downward. A slip would send you into the abyss. I held onto the chain and concentrated on each step, taking care not to look down.

The focus on each small movement drove away my fear, even in places where there was no chain. When we reached Angel's Landing, a top-of-the-world spot with incredible panoramas, I realized something. I'm better at overcoming my fears now than before having cancer.

"I don't think you would have done this before," Moe said, wrapping me in his arms. He is probably right.

Fighting the Big C was quite a challenge. If I had not broken it down into smaller increments, it would have been overwhelming. So I learned to take things moment by moment, hour by hour, and day by day. It was hard at times, and scary, but one careful step at a time, I skirted the abyss and made it to the top of that mountain.

At the Angel's Landing summit, I saw the woman who had spoken to me posing atop a hoodoo (small rock formation) on one leg with her arms outstretched like the Karate Kid. I couldn't help admiring her fearlessness.

"Thanks for encouraging me," I said when she came down. "I'm really glad I came up here."

Next Thursday, on my first Thanksgiving post-cancer, I will be giving thanks for (among other things, like being cancer-free) the amazing physical recovery and improved mental toughness that allowed me to complete a climb like Angel's Landing.

Mother Knows Best

Monday, December 3, 2012

Last week, I had the great privilege to be with my mother on her seventy-fifth birthday. She lives near Palm Springs this time of year, soaking up rays with other "snowbirds" who flock in from colder parts of the country.

Like many of us, Mom still feels eighteen on the inside. Though she doesn't "look" seventy-five, the image in the mirror does not correspond with her idea of self. I feel the same way when viewing my own reflection, but here's a little something I've learned over the past year: Aging is good. *Not* aging is the bad thing.

Mom didn't spend much time lamenting her age, especially after we saw the Palm Springs Follies, a troupe of senior showgirls and guys who've still "got it" and love to "strut it." Old? Says who? Certainly not the seventy-seven-year-old chanteuse or the eighty-three-year-old tap dancer who owned the stage.

My mother is a shy person until you get to know her, and then the real Mary Ann appears. She tells funny stories, loves to laugh, and is an excellent listener. She's gifted in the common sense department. As my brother, Jay, and I walked along Palm Canyon Drive with our mother, I thought about the many things she's taught us by her example.

In her own quiet way, Mom has always "been there" for us. Many years ago, when my brother was down on his luck, she and her then-husband invited Jay and his young son to move in with them until things got better. This living arrangement lasted almost a year. Mom provided love, encouragement, shelter, and food to her son and grandson, and never complained.

Last winter, when I was being treated for cancer, she and her current partner, Ed, kept in close touch, and came out twice to help out. Mom was with me at the doctor's office the week after surgery, when they pulled tubes out of my chest and I almost passed out. I was so glad she had my back.

When my parents split up after nineteen years of marriage, my mother picked herself up, moved across the country, and started over. When her second husband died after thirteen years of marriage, she again regrouped and recreated her life. Time and again, she has shown us that life's hard knocks cannot defeat you if you keep getting back up.

A few years ago, Jay and I bought Mom a computer for her birthday. At the time, I joked that it was like giving a car to a cavewoman. Mom had never used a computer. We had to start from scratch, really pre-scratch, in teaching her computer skills. After the first hour, I feared we'd made a big mistake, but over the course of a weekend, she kept asking questions and practicing until she got it. I don't think I ever told her how impressed I was by her perseverance.

During my cancer battle, when I shared my doubts and fears with her, Mom kept saying, "Carrie, I know you are going to get through this and be just fine. It can't come out any other way." She said it with such confidence that I believed it, too.

My mother has done much to be proud of in her seventy-five years. I feel fortunate that she is still in my life, showing me the ropes and providing the love that only a mother can. Keep on reeling in the years, Mom.

Postscript: When I finished cancer treatment, my mother sent me a card. On the front was a drawing of a little bird that had just leapt over a hurdle. "Is there anything you can't do?" said the caption beneath the picture.

I opened the card and read:

"Dear Carrie,

"The answer to that question is NO!! You can even beat cancer! Love, Mom."

6 RECONSTRUCTION AND BEYOND

"Hope is the thing with feathers
That perches in the soul
And sings the tune without the words
And never stops at all."

—Emily Dickinson

Bye-Bye Barbie Boob

Wednesday, December 5, 2012

I have put off writing about the next step in my breast cancer saga, but it's happening tomorrow. At 6:30 a.m., I will arrive at Piper Outpatient Surgery Center for the second phase of breast reconstruction.

According to my doctor, the outpatient operation will last about ninety minutes. He will deflate and remove the saline-filled tissue expander that has sat like a rock on the left side of my chest since my mastectomy last February. Then he will insert a more comfortable and lifelike silicone implant that will feel less like Barbie's boob and more like Carrie's.

Next, the doctor will place a smaller silicone implant under the pectoral muscle beneath my right (good) breast. When he is finished, I should have a matched set.

For the record, I'm not a gal who ever fantasized about getting breast implants. I seriously considered skipping the whole reconstruction ordeal, and will be very unhappy if the good doctor over-sizes my new rack. That said, a normal-appearing chest would be nice. The doctor said he usually gets it right on the first try. Let's hope so.

From A to B

Wednesday, December 12, 2012

Following my surgery last Thursday, Moe read in the paperwork that I had received a one pound silicone implant on the left (mastectomy) side of my chest, and a half pound implant on the right side. "That means you are twice as big as before," he said.

"No," I replied, looking down. "Really?" "Big" is not a word ever used to describe my bust line, and still won't be. The "girls" may have jumped from A to B, a modest change that I can accept. More importantly, they are now on an even plane and well-matched size-wise. Six days out, it appears this surgery was a success.

At a follow-up visit yesterday, the plastic surgeon's assistant reminded me that I am not out of the woods. Any activity that raises blood pressure or strains the chest area could cause bleeding and result in further surgery. She advised minimal walking, lifting, housework, and no sudden upper-body movements over the next few weeks. I didn't say a word about my three-and-a-half-mile walk in the park that morning, but she could tell from the look on my face that I already had broken most of the rules.

To impress upon me that rule breaking can have dire consequences, the doctor's assistant told me about the patient who called the office in a panic when her newly augmented breasts swelled dramatically. The swelling was due to bleeding set off by a vigorous sweeping of the kitchen floor three days after surgery. Then there was the gal who went snowboarding ten days after her procedure. "That was just stupid," the assistant said. Both women ended up back on the operating table.

Oddly, there was no cautionary tale about the woman who died of boredom and depression after three weeks of inactivity. I certainly don't intend to be *that* person, but I don't want another surgery, either. Going forward, I'm trying to be active enough to be happy, but not so active that I get myself in trouble.

For some reason, this is more challenging for me than the twelve hours of nausea that followed surgery, or the nightly muscle cramps resulting from being able to sleep only on my back. Like chemo and radiation, this too shall pass.

Postscript: My friend Lindsay, who endured a double-mastectomy and complicated reconstruction several years back, commented, "This post brought me right back to those days. Let me tell you, the first time I rolled over on my stomach at night (when allowed) was marvelous. Hope you are in for a super speedy recovery."

Following reconstruction, several weeks passed before I could comfortably sleep on my side, my preferred position. Almost a year later, I still don't stay long on the left side. Muscle cramps down that side of my back (usually after a long period of standing or hiking), and a frequent knot in the muscle between my neck and left shoulder, let me know that my body has not fully adjusted to the implant on the left. Physical therapy and a return to yoga might be needed.

Make that A to C

Monday, December 31, 2012

After my last post, I visited Victoria's Secret to be fitted for a new bra. There I learned that my new cup size is "C," not "B." I should have realized that from the look on my husband's face when he saw me after surgery.

You might think that Moe and I would be thrilled with this change, but we're conflicted. I told my surgeon I wanted to remain a small-breasted woman. My new bust line looks nice, and my clothes still fit (though not the bras), but I am now "medium" rather than "small." I can only conclude that "C" must seem small in my plastic surgeon's world. My husband, who liked me as I was, jokingly refers to my new boobs as "the strangers." I hope the nickname is short-lived.

A few times since surgery, I have wondered whether reconstruction was a mistake. From what I've read, it's normal to have such thoughts while enduring the discomforts of recovery. Though I really can't complain about the outcome of the surgery, I was surprised not only by the cup size, but also by the numbness in my healthy breast caused by nerve damage during placement of an implant on that side.

Since it's impossible to simulate fifty years of gravity, the surgeon placed an implant in the healthy breast to lift it up enough to match the reconstructed breast. According to a packet from the plastic surgeon's office, in 85 percent of cases in which nerves are damaged, feeling comes back in one to two years. These new breasts have reminded me, once more, that my body and life have been irrevocably changed by breast cancer.

Three-and-a-half weeks after surgery, I am back on the hiking trails, and any misgivings and sad feelings are fading. I know reconstruction was the right choice for me. I didn't want an empty space on the left side of my chest that would never let me forget about my cancer. I didn't want to feel self-conscious or worry about how clothes would fit. I didn't ask for size "C," but I'm not going to complain about it.

When life gives you lemons (or in my case, coconuts), make lemonade.

AFTERWORD

"When are you going to post again?"

"I miss your blog."

Such comments came to me via email and phone conversations in early 2013. I hadn't planned to end my blog on the last day of 2012, but as the New Year dawned I was still thinking about breast cancer all the time. It's a common problem among new survivors, and it gets in the way of moving on. I thought quitting the blog might be a good first step toward getting cancer out of my head.

Learning how to go forward from my illness as a wiser, stronger person, and not a victim, has been a priority ever since. In February 2013, I went on a women's empowerment weekend sponsored by the non-profit group Woman Within, hoping it would help me set a course toward new goals. As it turned out, the weekend had a different purpose. For a year-and-a-half, I'd been holding in feelings of sadness and loss due to cancer. Though I hadn't been aware of it, those feelings were possibly the biggest obstacle preventing me from moving forward. Woman Within provided a safe place to acknowledge my grief and release it, an important step in my emotional healing.

Perhaps that's when I realized that while I didn't want to spend my life obsessing over cancer, I couldn't just forget about it, either. There were too many reminders: my reconstructed left breast, which lacks nerve endings and nipple; the daily pill I take to keep cancer away; the vivid and sometimes haunting memories of treatment; and, of course, the possibility of recurrence always in the back of my mind. No, I couldn't pretend cancer didn't happen, nor did I want to ignore all that I learned from the experience.

I *could* turn a negative into a positive by being proactive against the disease. As a survivor, I have contributed to cancer charities, offered support and encouragement to anyone who needs it, and participated in the Susan G. Komen Race for the Cure and American Cancer Society's Relay for Life.

On the weekend of our first Relay for Life at our daughter's college (and our alma mater) in Los Angeles, my husband and I visited a college friend who was battling a recurrence of stomach/esophageal cancer. His was an aggressive type with limited treatment options. Doctors predicted he might live only six to eight months.

We left our friend's home saddened and with an altered perspective. How lucky I felt to have contracted a treatable breast cancer (serious though it was) instead of a form of the disease that is seldom cured. Relay for Life seemed more important than ever. Our buddy passed away at age fifty-seven, only two months after we visited, leaving behind a wife and two young children.

I want to be involved in cancer fundraisers for the rest of my life, especially those that prioritize research and help the less fortunate afford treatment, because cancer ravages lives and we need cures. Fighting back, even in small ways, feels good and gives me hope for the future.

My go-round with breast cancer taught me just how badly I wanted a future. If I got one, I resolved to make the best of it, which begged the question, "Once you get through this, how will you live differently?" During chemo, I started looking for answers, observing other people's lives to determine who was happy, who wasn't, and why. The research is ongoing and influences the way I now live.

Worries, including some that were not my own, used to make my stomach churn daily. How might I smooth things over between family members who weren't getting along? When should I stop loaning money to a relative perpetually in financial crisis? How could I please everyone all of the time (impossible!)? The fretting didn't help anyone and actually did me harm. Post-cancer, I'm less of a worrier. Some problems you can't fix, even if you'd like to. I do what I can and let them go.

Along the same lines, I don't care as much about what other people think. The house doesn't have to be perfect when guests come over. I'm more satisfied with and appreciative of what I have. I accept family members as they are, and am less inclined to be anyone's critic.

When my competitive nature makes me upset that I am slower than I used to be when hiking uphill or riding my bike, a new inner voice, that of a cancer survivor, reminds me, "You are fortunate to be able to do these activities at all." Yes I am. Life is good.

My husband and I are tackling our bucket list now, in our fifties, rather than waiting for some ideal time in the future. We have responsibilities, but try to have fun every day. Happiness is simpler than I thought, and, oftentimes, I believe it is a choice.

Despite my determination to live in the moment and let go of worries, I still face off with "The Monster," my moniker for the fear of death, at vulnerable moments. Recently, on a South American nature tour, my husband and I met some older folks who showed us what it means to thumb your nose at The Monster.

One of them, eighty-one-year-old Spike, spent many hours toting forty pounds of camera gear over his shoulder. Though he breathed heavily as we traipsed through the cloud forest and across volcanic islands, he never complained or seemed to slow down. A gifted photographer, he took great care in composing pictures of wildlife. The results seemed worthy of National Geographic.

After learning I was a recent cancer survivor, Spike's wife Judy confided that her husband was battling lung cancer. "He lost half a lung a few years ago, and now the cancer has metastasized to his shoulder," she said.

Weeks before the trip, doctors told the couple that Spike didn't have long to live, and to contact Hospice. In a last-ditch long shot, they ran a test to see whether Spike's might be a rare form of lung cancer that responds to a new treatment—a pill he could carry with him while traveling abroad. Turns out he was among the lucky 1.5 percent with this type of lung cancer. Spike received a prescription that put him in remission, and the couple packed for their fifty-fifth anniversary trip to Ecuador.

Without knowing it, Spike and Judy delivered a message to me: "This is how you do it."

Despite age and adversity, they were too busy living to worry about dying. I want to be like them—and to someday be their age.

I hope there are many more outdoor adventures in my future. Completing the rim-to-rim-to-rim hike in the Grand Canyon shortly after treatment gave me the confidence to accompany my husband on a ninety-mile backpacking trip across the Sierra Nevada on the John Muir Trail the following summer. Next year, Moe and I are considering a trek up 19,340-foot Mount Kilimanjaro, Africa's highest point. That would be special, no doubt, but it will be hard to top the Grand Canyon crossing of 2012. I am glad that Moe and I are no longer putting off the things we want to do until a more convenient time in the future. My illness taught us that there really is no time like the present.

Years ago, an acquaintance of mine was diagnosed with breast cancer while in her forties. The first among my circle of friends to get the disease, she was tight-lipped about her condition. What little she revealed was passed around in whispers, as if breast cancer were cause for shame. Many of us offered moral support, and would like to have done more, but didn't know what she needed.

Like my friend, some breast cancer patients prefer to go it alone. They dread the sympathy, speculation and stares that inevitably follow disclosure of a cancer diagnosis. Some fear it will be a distraction in the workplace. They don't want to talk about the difficulty of treatment or their feelings about it. Not wanting to appear weak, they politely reject offers of help. These people are brave and stoic, but I don't know how they do it.

While I respect each person's right to deal with breast cancer on her own terms, I'm glad that the diagnosis is no longer something patients feel they must hide. Being open about having cancer helped me immeasurably. Writing and talking about the experience allowed me to process what was going on and examine my feelings. It gave friends and family a window into my world, and invited them along for the ride. Because I had partners in my cancer journey, I seldom felt isolated or depressed.

Looking back, I have no regrets about sharing practically everything. No one ever complained I was providing too much information, even after I wrote about constipation. I only got complaints when the blog posts became infrequent, and when I finally ended them.

For me, openness was the right decision. I drew strength from the community of people who followed my progress and offered support in a hundred different ways. They bolstered me through treatment and helped me become a survivor.

Could I have done it on my own? I think so, but it would have been a lot harder. Studies have shown that cancer patients and survivors who participate in support groups have better outcomes and longevity than those who don't. That doesn't surprise me. When something bad happens, it helps to talk about it. As long as you keep the self-pity and complaining in check, being open is part of a healthy emotional lifestyle.

Almost as soon as I stopped blogging, my husband began a campaign to get me to turn my cancer blog into a book, a process that has involved revisiting difficult events and emotions. I often found myself in tears, and sometimes had to put it aside for a while, but the job has gotten easier over time. I hope others facing breast cancer—including the 1 percent who are men—will benefit in some way from reading about my experience. They may be in for miles of bumpy road, but they can make it to the end, as I did—finding points of light to keep them going on the dark days, allowing themselves to see the humor in difficult situations, and continuing to put one foot in front of the other no matter what.

Soon this book will be done, and I can give my mystery novel another try. Or maybe I'll write something else. The important thing is to show up at the keyboard—and in life—to follow inspiration wherever it leads. After cancer, the sky's the limit.

CPSIA information can be obtained at www.ICGtesting.com
Printed in the USA
BVOW04s1953200514

353920BV00002B/2/P